Also by Michael Mosesson

FIBRINOGEN MEMOIRS: Journeys of a Clot Doctor
Published by IPBooks © 2020

FIBRINOGEN
W. Nieuwenhuizen, M.W. Mosesson, M de Matt, eds.
Annals of The New York Academy of Sciences. 936, 1-643, © 2001

MOLECULAR BIOLOGY OF FIBRINOGEN AND FIBRIN
M.W. Mosesson and R.F. Doolittle, eds.
Annals of The New York Academy of Sciences. 408:1-672, © 1983

FIBRINOGEN

MEMOIRS 2

*The Rise and Fall of The Fibrin
Cross-linking Controversy*

FIBRINOGEN MEMOIRS 2

The Rise and Fall of The Fibrin Cross-linking Controversy

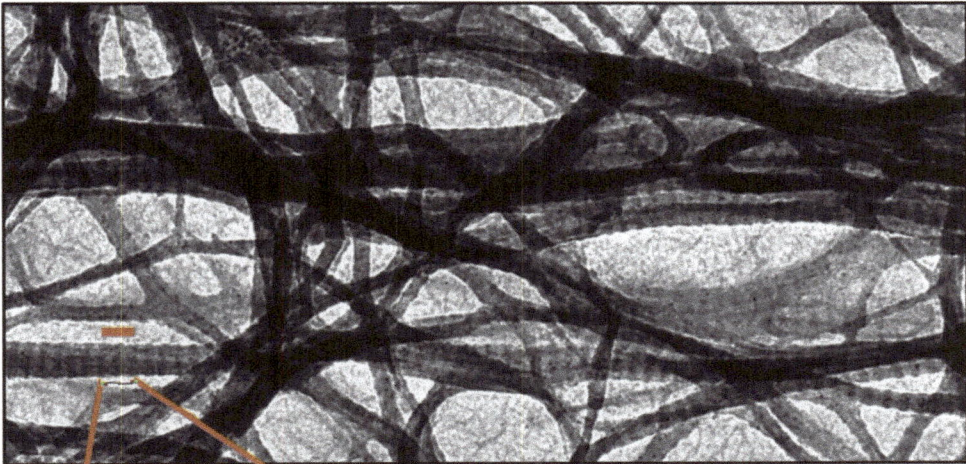

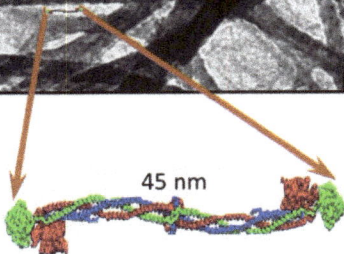

45 nm

MICHAEL W. MOSESSON

Fibrinogen Memoirs 2:
The Rise and Fall of the Fibrin Cross-linking Controversy
By Michael W. Mosesson

Published by IPBooks, Queens, NY
Online at: www.IPBooks.net

ISBN: 978-1-956864-04-5

Front cover design by Michael Mosesson
Back cover design by lisa roma
Editing, typesetting and layout design by lisa roma
Chapterhead Medieval caricature artwork by Roger Chen
All Photography copyright by Michael Mosesson
Scientific diagrams copyright by Michael Mosesson
Cover legend and graphic by Michael Mosesson

TABLE OF CONTENTS

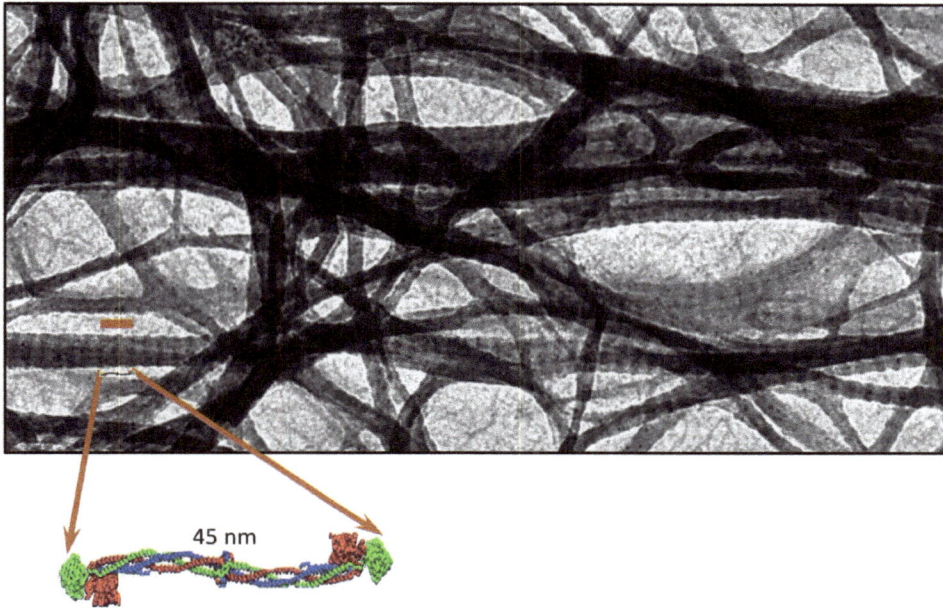

45 nm

Cover Legend

NETWORK FIBRILS AND FIBERS ARE COMPOSED OF FIBRIN MOLECULES

The Electron Micrograph (EM) on the cover shows a fibrin clot network magnified ~90,000 fold. Fibers display periodic banding at 22.5 nm intervals, equal to one-half the length of a fibrin molecule. The *bar* ▬ positioned over the fiber is 45 nm in length and spans exactly two bands. A fibrin molecule ▬ drawn to the scale of the EM, appears below the fiber. The drawing beneath the micrograph shows an ~11 fold enlargement of that fibrin molecule. (Drawing of the crystal structure of fibrinogen adapted from: Yang Z, Kollman JM, Pandi I, Doolittle RF. *Crystal Structure of Native Chicken Fibrinogen at 2.7Å Resolution.* Biochemistry 40:12515, 2001).

Dedication

This volume is dedicated to *Birger Blombäck* (1926-2008). His scientific contributions and discoveries were responsible for much of our current understanding of Fibrinogen structure, its purification, and its conversion to an insoluble polymer. Some of his work introduced methodologies and concepts that enhanced the precision of our experimental design and the validation of findings that we applied in arguing for a *transverse* cross-linking arrangement.

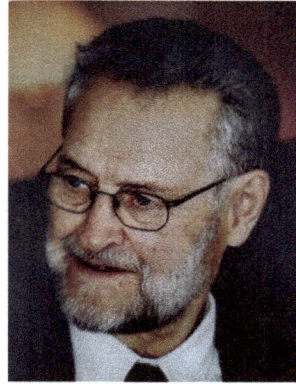

Birger's first significant publication [*Purification of Human and Bovine Fibrinogen.* Blombäck B, Blombäck M. *Arkiv Kemi* 10:415, 1956] introduced new methodology for purifying plasma fibrinogen. It employed an amino acid, glycine, in the buffers to adjust solubility and precipitability of heterogeneous plasma fibrinogen populations. Those procedures were the progenitor of methodologies for isolating and purifying previously unpurified and uncharacterized subfractions, one of which, 'Fraction I-9' or *Des /α-fibrinogen*, was of great value for the design of experimental protocols that could validate the existence of the *transverse* cross-linking arrangement.

Somewhat later in his career, his report that native Factor XIII induced gelation of fibrinogen [*Factor XIII Induced Gelation of Human Fibrinogen, An Alternative Thiol Enhanced Thrombin Independent Pathway.* Blombäck B, Procyk R, Adamson J, Hessel B. *Thromb Res* 37:613, 1985] was invaluable for conceptualizing how to produce cross-linked fibrinogen fibrils [13] as well as other thrombin independent cross-linked products.[1] That work also introduced the concept of an *in vivo* thrombin-independent role for Factor XIII.

During his long career, Birger published numerous studies on fibrinogen structure and its conversion to fibrin. He was the first to

---

[1] Birger wrote to me on a reprint of that article: *"To Michael with pleasant memories of friendship during years passed. This is my last work in the fibrinogen struggle. Yours Birger"*

identify the missense mutation that accounted for an amino acid substitution in a dysfibrinogen (*Fibrinogen Detroit*). He was prescient in recognizing the evolutionary implications of species differences between fibrinogen fibrinopeptides, an idea that he worked on with *Russ Doolittle* who further advanced the same concepts. These and other significant achievements were summarized in a memorial written by *Susan Lord* and *Agnes Henschen* [*J Thromb Haemostas* 7:908, 2009]. Birger summarized his career in a personalized article in 2006 [*Travels with Fibrinogen.* Blombäck B. *J Thromb Haemostas*. 4:1653, 2006].

We remained friends since first meeting socially in New York in 1975. Birger was at The New York Blood Center, and I was at SUNY-Downstate. One of Birger's qualities worth recalling was his humility and his willingness to listen to dissenting views and take them all into account, despite his opposing convictions. Unlike so many other famous people, he never pontificated, the epitome of a great scientist.

I saw him last in 2005 during a Baltic cruise when I visited him in Stockholm. We spent a joyful day at his home in Solna reminiscing and recalling 'good old days' that included amusing recollections of some of the protagonists mentioned in this book. I have an indelible recollection of him standing on the dock and waving wistfully to me as my ship departed.

Preface

By the end of 2019, after more than ten years' worth of frenetic writing, I had finally completed a 'final' draft of *Fibrinogen Memoirs,* and shortly afterward I placed it on a bookshelf for storage. By March of the following year, after having distributed a few printouts for review, I decided to upgrade and publish *Fibrinogen Memoirs*. By August 2020, I had formally signed off on the copy-edited version, secure in the knowledge that I had summarized many of my life's experiences, including the important scientific contributions.

During my research career, I authored and co-authored hundreds of peer-reviewed scientific articles, uncounted numbers of abstracts, edited and compiled several book editions, and a few textbook chapters. *Fibrinogen Memoirs* would be my first non-fiction narrative, a self-directed rendition of topics written in a format that did not require running the peer review 'gauntlet'.

My intent was to be rigorous in preserving historical accuracy, including precise documentation and description of personal and scientific experiences. I took this as an opportunity to reveal the human aspects of my experiences. It was also an opportunity to minimize the number of literature citations in favor of ones that were more topical. The goal was to provide sufficient background and detailed information to achieve clarity and comprehensibility for topically and scientifically informed readers as well as those who lacked an extensive background on the subjects at hand.

Regardless of whether I succeeded in those efforts, at first, I had no plans to revisit any subject that had been covered in that volume. That plan changed shortly after *Fibrinogen Memoirs* had gone 'to press', and after I had read a 2017 review article by *Litvinov* and *Weisel*. Their article covered recent advances on the biomechanical properties of fibrin polymers and their interpretation of these studies in terms of the presumed polymer structure of fibrin.

I had already covered critical aspects of that subject in chapter VI. It was entitled, *'Fibrin, The Perfect Bioelastomer'*. I had devoted most of the narrative to a description and analysis of the existing controversy about the positioning of cross-linked γ chains in an assembled fibrin clot. Two possible cross-linking arrangements had been promulgated, *transverse* or *longitudinal*, and only one of them could be correct.

After considering the functional properties of each possible cross-linking arrangement, I confidently proposed that there was an *ineluctable* association between *transverse* positioning of γ chain cross-links and the *elasticity* of a cross-linked fibrin clot. I extended that reasoning by offering that *longitudinal* positioning of cross-links could not account for fibrin's known perfect *elasticity*, since stretching such a configuration would instead result in *inelastic clot deformation (i.e., viscous deformation) which is* a feature of *non-cross-linked* clots but not of those that have been *cross-linked*.

Eberhard Selmayr was the first to propose *transverse* positioning of cross-linked γ chains in 1985; he supported that idea with another report in 1988. In the years following those reports, what had started as a disagreement grew into a full-blown, often contentious *controversy* that culminated a few years later in formal 'Debate' articles that were published in 2004 by two of the protagonists, *John Weisel,* and myself. Both articles and the follow up 'Rebuttals' were comprehensive documents that outlined the perceived strengths of their stated position and the weaknesses of the alternative arrangement.

Those articles marked the end of the formal publications devoted to the controversy, since following their appearance there were no written responses from the scientific community, and no new experimental reports bearing on either hypothesis. During the interval between 2004 and 2020 when *Fibrinogen Memoirs* was published, the subject had become dormant and not even one suggestion that such a controversy had ever existed.

To backtrack somewhat, by 2010 I had become discouraged by that dormancy, and withdrew completely from all matters relating to the fibrin cross-linking issue. Instead, I pursued other investigative interests until 2020 when I came across the 2017 *Litvinov/Weisel* article. That article served as a wakeup call that ended my non-participation. I soon filled the knowledge gap that had been created by my decade-long absence. It became clear that in place of a cross-linking controversy, the *longitudinal* cross-linking arrangement had become dogma and the concept of a *transverse* arrangement was non-existent. That turn of events was difficult to understand, and even more difficult to accept. Most importantly, it was accompanied by the realization that despite impressive advances in measuring biomechanical properties of fibrin, there could be no useful advances in explaining the relationship between fibrin polymer structure and fibrin's functional properties. Following that epiphany, I set out to write this present volume, *Fibrinogen Memoirs–The Rise and Fall of the Cros-linking Controversy*. My goal was to resurrect the controversy that had disappeared, with the hope that restoration of the underlying concepts would eventually lead to a sustainable explanation for the elasticity of cross-linked fibrin.

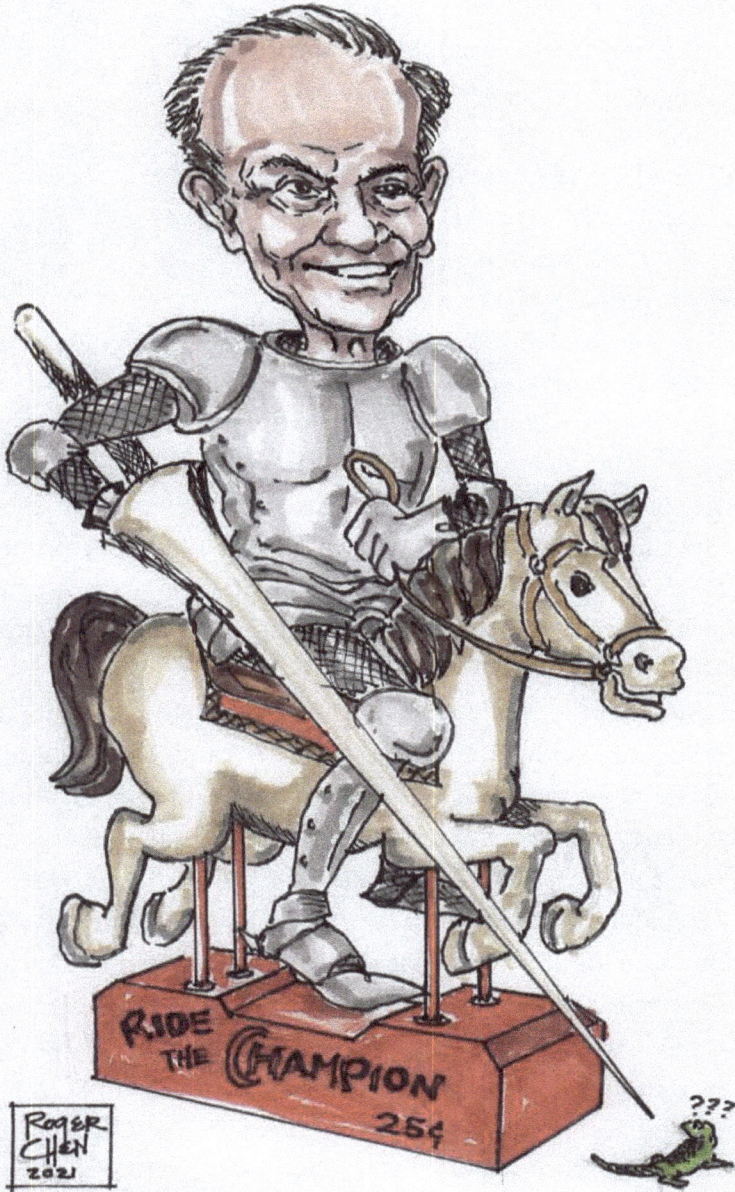

Chapter 1

Michael Mosesson

Michael Mosesson and The Controversy

M*ichael Mosesson*, one of the protagonists in the Controversy, was raised and educated in New York, graduating from Brooklyn College (BS, 1955) and subsequently from The State University of New York-Downstate Medical Center (SUNY; MD, 1959). He spent one year at Boston City Hospital in Medical Residency, followed by three-years of military service in The US Public Health Service (USPHS) at The Division of Biologics Standards (DBS) in Bethesda, Maryland. At DBS he quickly developed expertise in *Fibrinogen*, the soluble, circulating blood protein that self-assembles to form *fibrin clots* after being activated by Thrombin to *Fibrin*. He applied that new knowledge to help resolve an existing problem concerned with accurately measuring the several components found in commercially produced *Fibrinolytic* agents that were being considered for licensure by an agency that eventually became a subsidiary of the Food and Drug Administration (FDA).

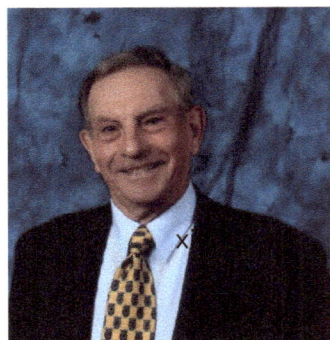

The success he enjoyed while serving in the USPHS at DBS engendered an intense and enduring research and clinical interest in *fibrinogen*. To advance that goal he relocated to St Louis, MO, to complete Medical Residency training at Barnes Hospital, accompanied by an offer from *Professor Sol Sherry* to join and participate in the activities of his *Fibrinolysis* research and clinical group called The Enzymology Section. During a four-year period with that group, he advanced his knowledge of *Clinical Fibrinolytic* therapy and also published several research studies concerned a new subject, *Circulating Fibrinogen Catabolites.*

After that highly productive period he returned to SUNY-DMC, where he headed an NIH funded Program Project Grant and rose to the Academic rank of Professor of Medicine and of Biochemistry. An important aspect of the move to New York was marriage to *Shirley Ann Mosesson* (née McDowell) and the subsequent birth of their three children *Matthew, Marni,* and *Aimee.*

After several years in New York, he took Sabbatical leave and moved to Paris, France, with his family for more than one year. While at Hôpital Beaujon in Clichy working with *Doris Ménaché* he was able to continue the activities of his New York research team while conducting studies of a French family with an inherited abnormality of fibrinogen (*dysfibrinogenemia*) that came to be known as 'Fibrinogen Paris I', as well as learning a valuable new technique, Electron Microscopy.

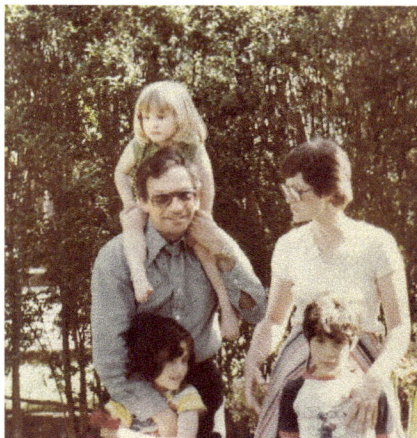

After returning to New York (1978), he further advanced his newly gained expertise in Electron Microscopy (EM) by collaborating with the Scanning Transmission Electron Microscopy (STEM) group at the Brookhaven National Laboratory (BNL) headed by *Joseph Wall*, who pioneered development of that technique. That collaboration was important particularly for Mosesson's studies related to *'The Fibrin Cross-linking Controversy'* and for determining the exact location of cross-linked γ chains in an assembled fibrin fibril.

After fourteen years in New York, he relocated to Milwaukee, Wisconsin, to be Director of the Research Division at Sinai Samaritan Medical Center (1981), a teaching campus of The University of Wisconsin School of Medicine (Madison). Shortly after his arrival in Milwaukee, he was invited to join the Scientific Advisory Committee (*Fachbeirat*) of *Gert Müller-Berghaus'* Hematology Research Group at Justus-Liebig Universität in Giessen, Germany. While in that capacity he met *Eberhard Selmayr* who was a Research Fellow in Müller-Berghaus' laboratory. At one of the Fachbeirat meetings (1985), Selmayr presented findings pointing to a *transverse* arrangement of cross-linked γ chains in assembled fibrin clots. At the time, the notion of a *transverse* cross-linking arrangement was a new concept for Mosesson, but he recognized its likely validity on experimental grounds and its potential physiological importance. Mosesson encouraged Selmayr to continue his investigations,

3

but when he chose to terminate his involvement in favor of his intended career in Veterinary Medicine, Mosesson decided to pick up 'the cudgel' on his own. That decision launched a prolonged and intense involvement in the cross-linking controversy that has now resulted in a second volume of *Fibrinogen Memoirs* dealing solely with the origins, history, and current disposition of the *Controversy*.

Mosesson maintained a focus during his career on bleeding and thrombotic disorders, fibrinogen, fibrinolysis, and other components of the blood coagulation system. His extensive experience related to blood coagulation make him well qualified to write this sequel of *Fibrinogen Memoirs*.

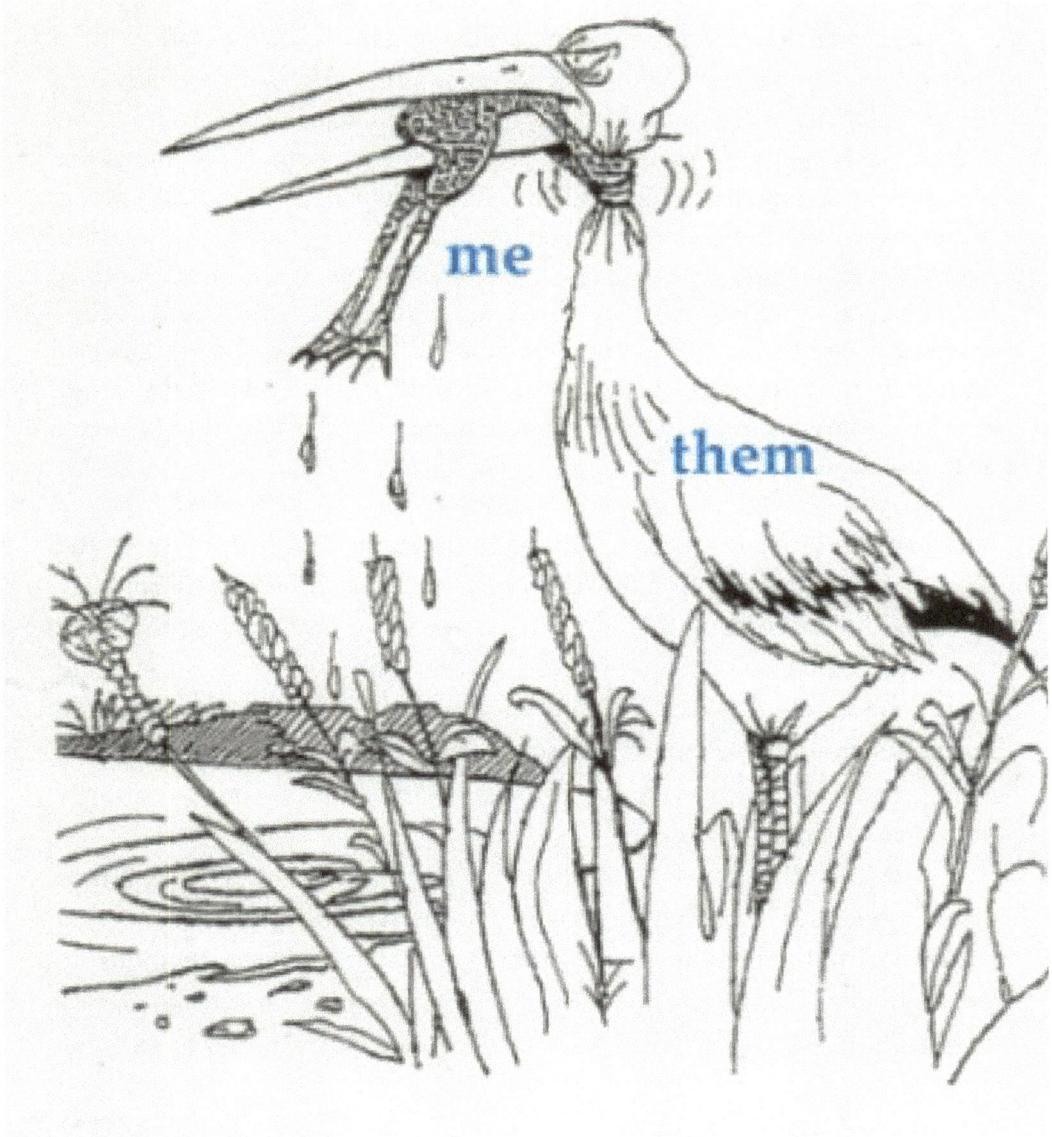

me

them

Don't Ever Give Up!

The Controversy Revisited

My first book, '*Fibrinogen Memoirs–Journeys of a Clot Doctor*', covered many previous scientific and personal journeys and adventures [1].

Chapter VI, '*Fibrin, The Perfect Bioelastomer*' [2],[2] dealt with a controversy focused on the location of cross-linked (*ligated*)[3] γ chains in a fibrin clot. The first substantive report on that subject appeared in 1981 and the last one that I am aware of, in 2002. Overwhelming evidence for a *transverse* arrangement had accumulated between 1986 and 2002 while arguments for the alternative arrangement, *longitudinal*, remained speculative and unsupported by evidence. Despite such an evidentiary imbalance, a consensus was never reached. The arguments for and against reached a zenith in 2004 with publication of the '*Cross-linking Debates*' crafted by the two main adversaries at the time, *John Weisel* and me. These articles and the *rebuttals* that followed summarized the available evidence and rationales.

Another subject related to cross-linking was the relationship between the locations of cross-linked γ chains in a fibrin polymer, and their capacity to account for the *elasticity* of a stretched fibrin clot. Although proof for that relationship was lacking, at the time I reasoned that only a *transverse* cross-linked γ chain arrangement could support such behavior. A *longitudinal* bond arrangement, were it to exist, could not support such a property. Instead, strain imposed on a *longitudinal* arrangement would result in *viscous deformation*, a well-known property of non-cross-linked fibrin.

It is well established that *elasticity* is a property of cross-linked fibrin clots, but it is *not* a property of non-cross-linked clots. That realization led me to infer that there was an *ineluctable* relationship between fibrin elasticity and '*transverse*' positioning of cross-linked γ chains [2]. I was aware that more evidence would be needed to nail that

---

[2] Here is a link to Chapter VI for readers wishing to pursue a more detailed understanding of events: https://1drv.ms/w/s!Aq41MDElk2zZtU0oyWuiXtT3aYuV?e=YStodz

[3] John Ferry used the word '*ligation*' to describe the fibrin *cross-linking* process. I agree with that terminology, but '*cross-linking*' has been in use for so long that I opted to stay with that term in this publication.

down. As it turned out, the 'necessary' additional evidence emerged after the Debates.

During the sixteen years that followed the 2004 Debate articles, no new evidence dealing with the contested cross-linking arrangements appeared. That was not surprising since virtually all the experimental approaches that might have shed new light on the subject had been explored. What did surprise me about what occurred in that period was the total abandonment of the *transverse* cross-linking scheme, and substitution by dogmatic assumption of the *longitudinal* arrangement.

In 2010, *Martin Guthold's* group published a report on the mechanical properties of single fibrin fibers [3]. In modeling their findings, they ignored the cross-linking controversy entirely and simply assumed that a *longitudinal* cross-linked bond arrangement existed in their fibers. They made no mention of the alternative arrangement. I voiced my concerns in a '*Letter-to-the-Editor*' entitled: *Short by One Mechanism* [4]. The 'Letter' resulted in a brief exchange of emails between Martin and myself but nothing came of it. I was deeply disappointed by that oversight and, shortly afterward, I curtailed my interest and activities in the fibrin cross-linking issue for a decade.

My interest in this subject was renewed in August of 2020, almost immediately after I had signed off on the final proofing of *Fibrinogen Memoirs*. An electronic message from *Elsevier* Publishing landed in my Inbox flagging a 2017 issue of *Matrix Biology* that was devoted to '*Fibrin and Fibrinogen*'. I downloaded several of the articles, among which was one entitled '*Fibrin Mechanical Properties and Their Structural Origins*' by *Litvinov* and *Weisel* [5]. After reading their review and the studies that they cited, I ended my decade-long leave-of-absence.

The *Litvinov* review covered, among various other related topics, studies of the biomechanical properties of fibrin. Most of these investigations assumed that the cross-linked γ chains in fibrin were arranged '*longitudinally*'; there was no recognition that a controversy had even existed. *Longitudinal* cross-linking was now *dogma* and the *transverse* arrangement had been relegated to the 'Endangered Species' list, a virtual *Myth*! My chapter in *Fibrinogen Memoirs*, '*Fibrin, The Perfect Bioelastomer*', although still useful, would need updating and reinforcement.

In writing the sequel, I hoped to *unearth* (pun intended) how *interment* and *mythification* had come about and if possible, determine how and why a lively, unresolved controversy had become so marginalized. I also wanted to draw attention one more time to evidence for a *'transverse' cross-linking'* arrangement. The only way to achieve that goal was for me to write another volume of *Fibrinogen Memoirs*.

I had no idea whether the approach I had chosen would succeed but like the legendary *Don Quixote*, I resolved to try.

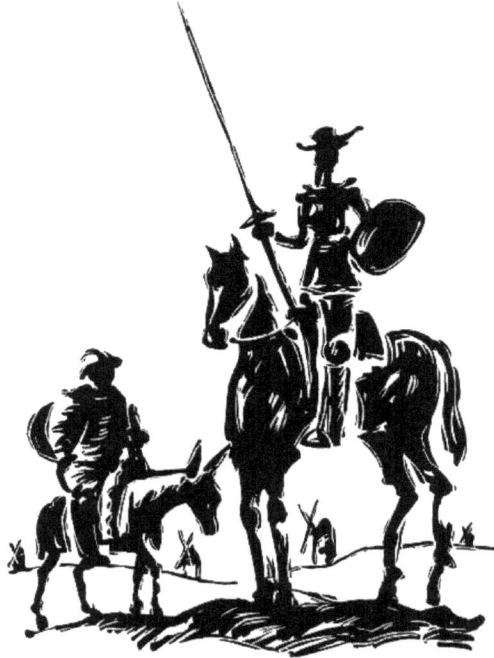

Chapter 3
Fibrinogen Conversion to Fibrin, Fibril Assembly, and The Clot Network

This chapter contains information, notations, symbols, and terminology that can be used to gain an understanding of fibrinogen structure, its conversion to fibrin, fibrin self-assembly to form double-stranded fibrils, and the *transverse* positioning of the carboxy-terminal γ chains in the fibril (Figure 1). This information will serve as a useful roadmap and guide in later sections for understanding the controversy that existed about an alternative arrangement of the carboxy-terminal γ chains, *longitudinal*. The controversy over the location of cross-linked γ chains in a fibrin polymer is the main subject of this book and will be addressed in detail later.

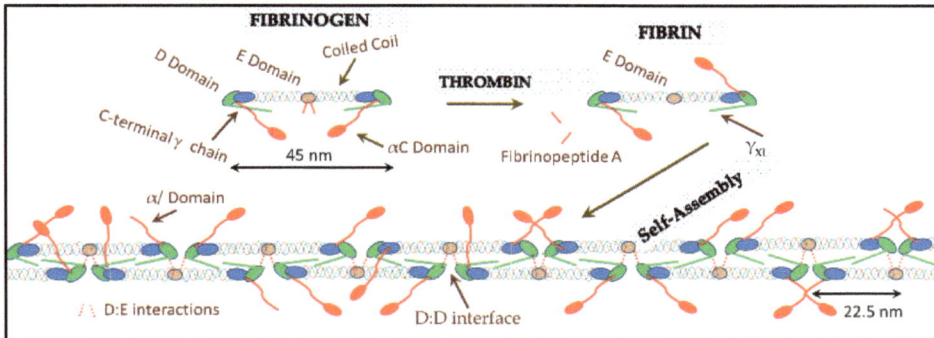

Figure 1. *Drawing of a **Fibrinogen** molecule (upper left) illustrating its major domains. The D and E Domains of each molecule are connected through coiled coils* ∿∿∿. ***Fibrin** (upper right) is generated from fibrinogen when **thrombin** cleaves two **Fibrinopeptides A** /\ from each E* **Domain** ⊙ *to expose two E Domain polymerization sites. Fibrin molecules, each 45 nm in length, undergo self-assembly through non-covalent interactions* ⸫ *between constitutive sites in* **D** *Domains and fibrin* **E** *Domain sites. The* **D:E** *interactions drive the formation of double-stranded fibrils in a half-staggered molecular arrangement. Fibrils display a periodicity of 22.5 nm that is exactly one half the length of a fibrin molecule.*

Fibrinogen is the circulating precursor of *Fibrin*. Each molecule is composed of two sets of chains termed Aα (red), Bβ (blue), and γ (green), that are bound together in the central region by covalent disulfide bonds that form the 'dimeric' E Domain,(⊙ The three chains form 'coiled coils' that connect the D and E Domains. The carboxy-terminal regions of γ

9

chains (⟋) emerge from each D Domain, as illustrated above. Cross-linking sites termed γ_{XL} , are located near its tail end.

   Fibrin is generated after cleavage and release of two peptides, termed *Fibrinopeptides A*(/\ ) from the E Domain of fibrinogen, exposing polymerization sites that then form intermolecular non-covalent bridges with opposing D Domains ('D:E'). These interactions drive self-assembly of a half-staggered array of linearly aligned fibrin molecules that form double-stranded fibrils displaying 22.5 nm periodicity, a distance amounting to half the length of a fibrinogen molecule, 45 nm.

   Structures containing the carboxy-terminal regions of Aα chains, are termed 'αC domains' (⌒), and emanate from the D Domains, as illustrated. A shortened *in vivo* derived proteolytic derivative, α/ lacks the segments that participate in FXIII-catalyzed cross-linking to form *'α-polymers'*.[4]

The Fibrin Clot Network (Figure 2)

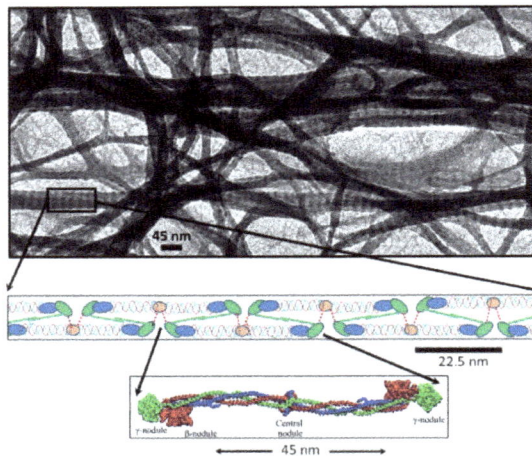

Figure 2. *Structures comprising a fibrin clot network.* The Electron Micrograph at the top shows a fibrin clot network magnified ~90,000 times (*Bar* = 45 nm). Network fibers, composed of multiple laterally aligned fibrils, show periodic banding (e.g., *within the rectangle*). Each fibril consists of end-to-end aligned fibrin molecules forming two parallel strands arrayed in a half-staggered arrangement that confers 22.5 nm periodicity (*i.e., the*

---

[4] All Aα chains in plama fibrinogen subfractions like 'Fraction I-9' (*Des /α-Fibrinogen*) are truncated and lack the cross-linking sites that exist only in the missing carboxy-terminal segments. We used this subfraction when formation of cross-linked 'α-polymers' might have complicated our interpretations.

drawing beneath the micrograph, enlarged ~9-fold). The *lower drawing* shows the crystal structure of fibrin(ogen) enlarged -2-fold over the molecules in the drawing above it. (Adapted from Yang Z, Kollman JM, Pandi I, Doolittle RF. *Crystal Structure of Native Chicken Fibrinogen at 2.7Å Resolution.* Biochemistry 40:12515, 2001).

Chapter 4
Timeline of Events

1973– *Russ Doolittle* [6] speculates that carboxy-terminal regions of γ chains emerge from D Domains as short squiggly filaments that interact with neighboring filaments in an end-to-end alignment. There is no evidence to support his conjecture, and as yet, no alternative suggestions.

1981– *Walter Fowler* [7] identifies cross-linked D-dimers ●━● in electron microscopic studies of fibrin degradation products and proposes that the observed end-to-end alignment of D Domains reflects the cross-linking arrangement in fibrin fibrils. This was the opening gambit in the evolving controversy.

1985– *Eberhard Selmayr* et al. [8] show that Factor XIII catalyzed cross-links forming between fibrinogen and bead-immobilized fibrin are positioned *transversely*. The controversy begins!

1988– *Selmayr et al.* [9] report their findings on electron microscopic investigations of urea-dissociated fibrin fibers. These results bolster their earlier conclusions.

1989– *Mosesson et al.* [10] identify higher ordered cross-linked *trimeric* and *tetrameric* γ chains after prolonged incubation with Factor XIII, findings that are consistent with *transverse* positioning of γ chains in fibrin fibrils!

1993– *Weisel et al.* [11] report finding covalently linked D-dimers ●━● in digests of cross-linked fibrin that had been processed prior to imaging in *acetic acid* solutions that *dissociate* non-covalent bonds. Like Fowler before them, they mistakenly assumed that this observation provided evidence for a *longitudinal* bond arrangement in assembled fibrils. The controversy was now in full swing!

1995– To challenge Weisel's 1993 conclusions, *Siebenlist et al.* prepared cross-linked *D-fibrin-D* complexes and analyzed them by STEM [12]. Each outer D Domain of this complex was covalently connected to a fibrin D Domain by *cross-linked γ chains*. STEM images of *D-fibrin-D* specimens that had been deposited on a grid in physiological buffers (conditions that allowed non-covalent D:E interactions to take place), revealed a 'folded' configuration with the outer D Domains situated near the central fibrin E Domain . It followed from this configuration that the cross-linked γ chains connecting the D Domains to fibrin were positioned *transversely*! When these specimens were processed in acetic acid solutions (solvent conditions that disrupt D:E interactions), the *D-fibrin-D* complexes were unfolded and extended in a linear configuration (i.e., no fibrin E Domain contacts) . These findings refuted Weisel's earlier conclusions, but not surprisingly, did not end the controversy.

1995– *Mosesson et al.* [13] discovered that *fibrinogen* molecules that had been cross-linked in the presence of Factor XIII, formed half-staggered *double-stranded fibrils* and *laterally associated* fibers displaying the same 22.5 nm periodicity as found in fibrin fibrils. *Fibrinogen* fibrils had formed solely **because** of *transverse* positioning of cross-linked γ chains!

1996– The pencil diagram in *John Ferry's* letter to Mosesson leads to a new undertanding of an *ineluctable* association between *transverse* positioning of cross-linked γ chains and fibrin *elasticity*!

1997– *Doolittle et al.* [15] reported on the structure of crystallized D fragments he called *'double-D'*. The cross linked γ chain segments (dotted line) connecting the D Fragments was *not* visualized. These structures were taken as proof for a *longitudinal* arrangement of cross-linked γ chains in fibrin fibrils, further confounding the Controversy.

1998– *Veklich et al.* [16] reported on cross-linking fibrinogen molecules that had been assembled on a fibrin fragment E template. They used an acetic acid solution to dissociate non-covalent bonds in these samples and found single-stranded linearly aligned cross-linked fibrinogen fibrils and *unbound* E fragments. Their conjecture was that these observations provided evidence for a *longitudinal* cross-link arrangement in fibrin. (*This turned out to be Weisel's last experimental contribution to the controversy.*)

1998– *Mosesson et al.* [19] labeled cross-linking sites in fibrinogen and fibrin γ chains with cadaverine that had been tagged with an electron dense gold particle, Au11, and readily detectable by STEM. Most gold particles were situated between the D and E domains, a finding indicating that carboxy-terminal regions of γ chains tend to be situated in positions that make them available for *transverse* cross-linking!

2000– *Yakovlev et al.* [20] demonstrated that the middle β-strand of a five-stranded antiparallel β-sheet in the γ module of the D Domain could be pulled out without disrupting the overall γ module structure. These findings led to their *'pull out'* hypothesis that illustrated how unfolding of these structures could span the distance required for *transverse* cross-linking to take place!

2000– *Siebenlist et al.* reported results of a cross-linking experiment that exploited size differences between fibrinogen γA and γ' chains [23]. They mixed radioactively labeled γA-γ' *fibrin* with non-radioactive γA-γA *fibrinogen* , then cross-linked the fibrin/fibrinogen mixture and determined the distribution of radioactivity among the γ-dimers that had been produced. They found radioactive γA-γA and γA-γ' chains at a 1:1 ratio. Those were the cross-linked products expected for *transversely* positioned γ chains. The findings were categorically *inconsistent* with *longitudinally* positioned γ chain segments, since such an arrangement, had it existed, could *not* have formed radioactive γA-γA dimers, and in its place, monomeric radioactive γA- and γ' chains would have been found!

2002– *Mosesson et al.* [18], in response to the 1998 Veklich paper, reported their results of assembling fibrinogen in physiological buffers on a fibrin fragment E template (*des A-fragment E*), and then cross-linking them. STEM images revealed *double-stranded transversely cross-linked fibrils* similar to those previously found in *cross-linked fibrinogen fibrils (1995)*. These findings further validated *transverse* positioning of cross-linked γ chains in assembled fibrin fibrils!

2004– Mosesson and Weisel are invited by *Robert Ariens*, an Editor of JTH, to participate in a *Debate* on *Transverse* versus *Longitudinal* cross-linking, to be followed by rebuttal statements [24-27]. This event marked the zenith of the controversy.

2004 to 2020-

- Following the 2004 Debates, interest in the subject declined and no new research reports on the cross-linking issue appeared.
- **2005-***Mosesson* and *Weisel* begin a collaborative investigation based upon *Paul Bishop's* original idea. The experiment could provide an unambiguous distinction between *longitudinal* and *transverse* cross-linking arrangements. Just as the project was nearing completion (2006) Weisel discontinued his participation. Unfortunately, there were no reportable results!
- **2010-***Mosesson* withdraws from activities related to the cross-linking controversy, an absence that lasts a decade. *'Sleeping Beauty'* (aka *Mosesson*) awakens in **2020**, reassesses the situation, and begins writing a sequel to *Fibrinogen Memoirs*.

Chapter 5

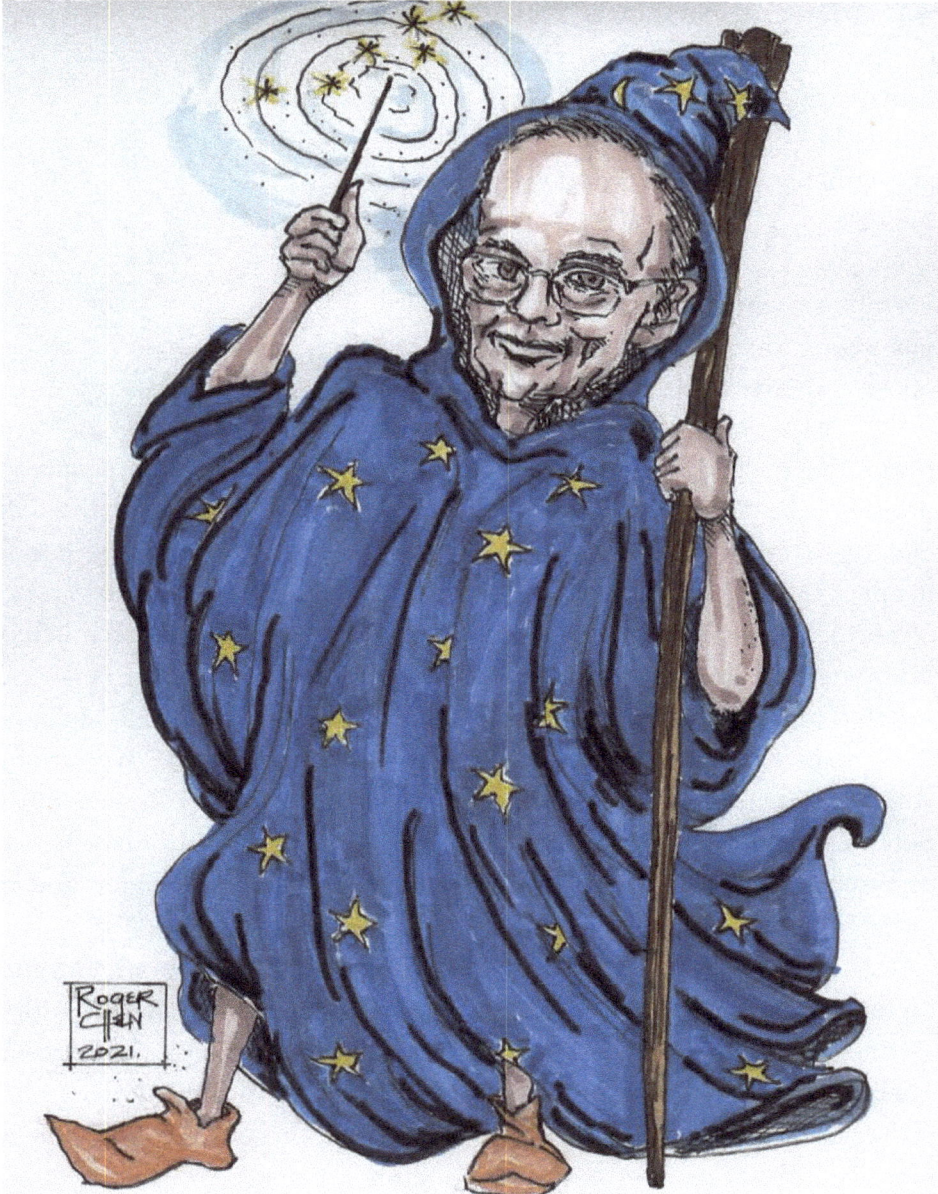

Russell F. Doolittle

Russell F. Doolittle

In the first volume of *Fibrinogen Memoirs*, I wrote disparagingly about Russ Doolittle's involvement in the cross-linking controversy. I portrayed him as single-minded with an unalterable and unjustifiable faith in the notion that cross-linked γ chains were arranged *longitudinally* in fibrin fibrils. Those narratives, while accurate at the time, are not nearly the complete story about this gifted and charismatic scientist.

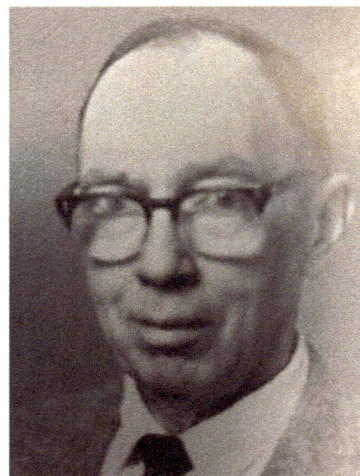

X-Ray crystallographic analyses of fibrin Fragment D and what Russ called 'Double-D' (aka, *D dimer*), provided the fodder for his unshakable convictions. Acquiring the data and the subsequent analyses required considerable effort and expertise on his part. Subsequently, he extended the same expertise to obtain crystals of fibrinogen molecules. All were meritorious studies, as was so much of his other work, but unfortunately, they were overinterpreted.

I argued repeatedly and vigorously with him that the crystallized D Domain structures from which he drew his conclusions, were not a valid representation of the situation that exists in a cross-linked fibrin polymer. To no avail! He was also dismissive of EM studies that showed precisely where these structures were to be found in fibrinogen and in fibrin fibrils.

He also argued that the cross-linking site in the carboxy-terminal region of a fibrin γ chain could not extend sufficiently to interact with a second γ chain in a *transverse* position, his so-called 'distance' argument. That notion was challenged by the *Yakovlev/Medved* studies showing how this region could be 'pulled out' reversibly from its position in the γ-module of the D domain, to span the required distance.

These descriptions are not a representation of Doolittle's other achievements or his other scientific contributions, to say nothing of his legendary oratory skills. In the following paragraphs, I will consider work that led to some of those contributions, including some memorable personal interactions.

Russ became interested in blood clotting while he was in the doctoral program at the Department of Biological Chemistry at Harvard Medical School under the aegis of *J. Lawrence Oncley*, and he stayed with that subject for his entire career. After obtaining his degree in 1961 he migrated to *Birger Blombäck's* laboratory at the Karolinska Institute in Sweden on a post-doctoral fellowship where Blombäck was investigating the amino acid sequences of the 'fibrinopeptides' that are cleaved and released from mammalian fibrinogen by thrombin. Blombäck realized that these sequences could reveal evolutionary relationships of these species. Doolittle pounced on this idea and with Blombäck they extended their inquiry to construct phylogenetic trees yielding important information about speciation over periods of millions of years. Later, Doolittle further expanded his studies to include primate fibrinopeptides, leading to a better understanding of the relationship between chimpanzees and humans. His efforts to produce a 'molecular clock' continued to drive his inquiries and were important contributors to the burgeoning field of molecular evolution. This seminal work no doubt contributed to his election to the National Academy of Sciences in 1984.

To further expand his own investigations of molecular evolution, he undertook studies of the structure and amino acid sequence of *Lamprey fibrinogen*, a member of the chordate phylum that was most distant from mammals. In 1993, he offered to collaborate with me in an investigation of the ultrastructure of Lamprey fibrinogen and fibrin. I enthusiastically agreed to this, and he soon provided me with Lamprey plasma, purified Lamprey fibrinogen, and Lamprey thrombin. The imaging analyses were completed the following year. I sent Russ a detailed report and proposed publishing the results. Inexplicably at the time, he declined to pursue that inquiry any further and our report was never published[5]

---

[5] Russ declining to publish these results might have been related to the fact that during that same period we were in adversarial positions on the cross-linking issue. In lieu of a publication, I placed a comprehensive draft of this work in the *Mosesson Library* at the Blood Research Institute of the BloodCenter of Wisconsin.

Concomitant with his Lamprey investigations, Russ explored how the fibrinogen molecule might have evolved as a covalently linked dimeric molecule composed of three pairs of homologous chains (α, β, γ). Several years later he discovered from genomic analyses of the protochordate, *Ciona Intestinalis*, the Sea Squirt, that there was a DNA message for a protein similar to mammalian fibrinogen although there were no thrombin cleavable sites to be found. Furthermore, Sea Squirt hemolymph does not clot. In Doolittle's own words, "*it was like an anthropologist stumbling across a veritable 'Lucy' of molecular antiquity*". Based upon that sequence homology he was able to construct a hypothetical molecular model of Sea Squirt *'protofibrinogen'* that closely resembled mammalian fibrinogen (see bottom of figure below).

To better represent these remarkable achievements, I prepared a composite illustration (Figure) containing previously unpublished EM images of rotary shadowed Human (*first row, middle*) and Lamprey

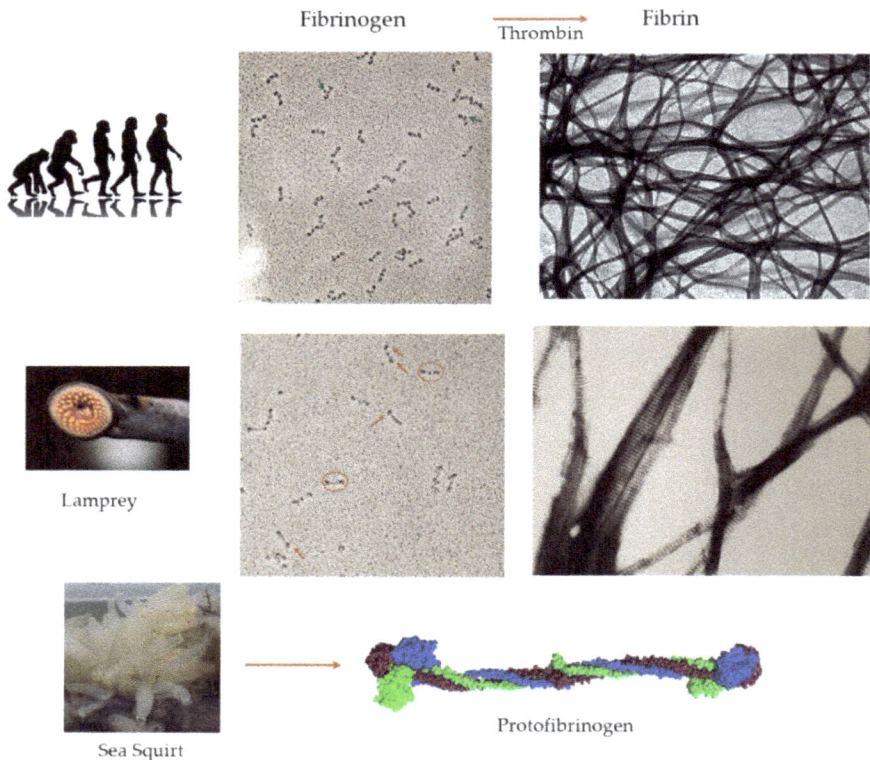

Fibrinogen   → Thrombin   Fibrin

Lamprey

Sea Squirt   →   Protofibrinogen

Figure. *A comparison of Human and Lamprey Fibrinogen molecules and the fibrin networks produced following thrombin cleavage and fibrin self-assembly (Rows 1 and 2). Lamprey fibrin fibers are considerably thicker than the human fibrin fibers formed under the same solvent conditions. The 22.5 nm periodicity of Lamprey fibrin, like human, corresponds to one half the length of a fibrinogen molecule. The bottom row shows Doolittle's model of a Sea Squirt Protofibrinogen molecule [Doolittle RF, J Innate Immun 4:219-222, 2012].*

fibrinogen (*second row, middle*), and their respective fibrin networks (*rows 1 and 2, right*). The *bottom row* shows a Sea Squirt (*left*) and Russ's proposed model of Sea Squirt '*protofibrinogen*'. (Compare this model with the image of a crystallized chicken fibrinogen molecule on the cover page.)

Lamprey fibrinogen molecules, like those of mammalian origin, are elongated 45 nm, trinodular structures [*ovals, middle row*]. Commonly there is another globular shaped structure about the size of a D Domain [*arrows, middle row*] which tends to overlap or be located near outer D Domains. This 'extra' domain corresponds to the structure predicted from its DNA-derived amino acid sequence.

Those were not *Doolittle's* only noteworthy scientific achievements. These include his discovery of *reciprocal covalent bridging* of cross-linked fibrin γ chains, his contributions toward determination of the amino acid sequence of human and Lamprey fibrinogen, his analyses of crystals of human D Domain and cross-linked D dimers, and chicken fibrinogen. Altogether, this body of work reflects the lifelong accomplishments of an imaginative, focused, and productive scientist.

Russ and I had some personal interactions worth recalling: In 1974, he was Moderator of a session on '*Fibrinogen Structure*' at a Thrombosis and Hemostasis Conference that was held in Dallas, Texas. The subject matter involved an intensely debated argument at the time concerned with the structure of Fibrinogen. Main speakers were *Victor Marder, Andrei Budzynski, Patrick McKee, Birger Blombäck, John Finlayson* and me. John and I were defending what turned out to be the indefensible, although I did not accept that verdict at the time. Russ was erudite in moderating the conference in a well-balanced manner. At the end of the presentations and the intense discussion that followed, he ended the session by requesting that "*anyone who agreed with Finlayson and Mosesson, exit to the 'left'; those who did not, exit to the 'right'.*" I had a sinking feeling just then since only

John Finlayson, out of loyalty rather than conviction, exited with me on the left side of the auditorium. That episode is further detailed in Part 1 of *Fibrinogen Memoirs*, Chapter V.

In 1976, at a meeting of the International Society on Thrombosis and Hemostasis (ISTH) in Philadelphia we decided to have a 'run' together early one morning. We wound up inexplicably on a superhighway with no apparent way to find our way out. We both remembered that harrowing experience somewhat differently and both of us, fortunately, survived it.

In 1982, Russ and I organized and edited the proceedings of a New York Academy of Sciences conference on *'The Molecular Biology of Fibrinogen'*, a widely acclaimed and still cited publication.

We never settled our differences on the fibrin cross-linking controversy–his death in 2019 precluded that–but I never lost my respect and admiration for him, his keen intellect, and his sense of humor. His last communication to me, just weeks before his death was: *'I was very pleased to get your email! We do go back a long way. I, too, remember the run in Philadelphia, including clambering between railroad cars. And it has been great to be, like you, a "fibrinogen person". We were lucky to come on the scene when such problems could be attacked by individuals with small groups. Until recently I never appreciated the term "ravages of old age." But now I have encountered them. Thanks for your friendship over all these years. Russ.'*

Chapter 6

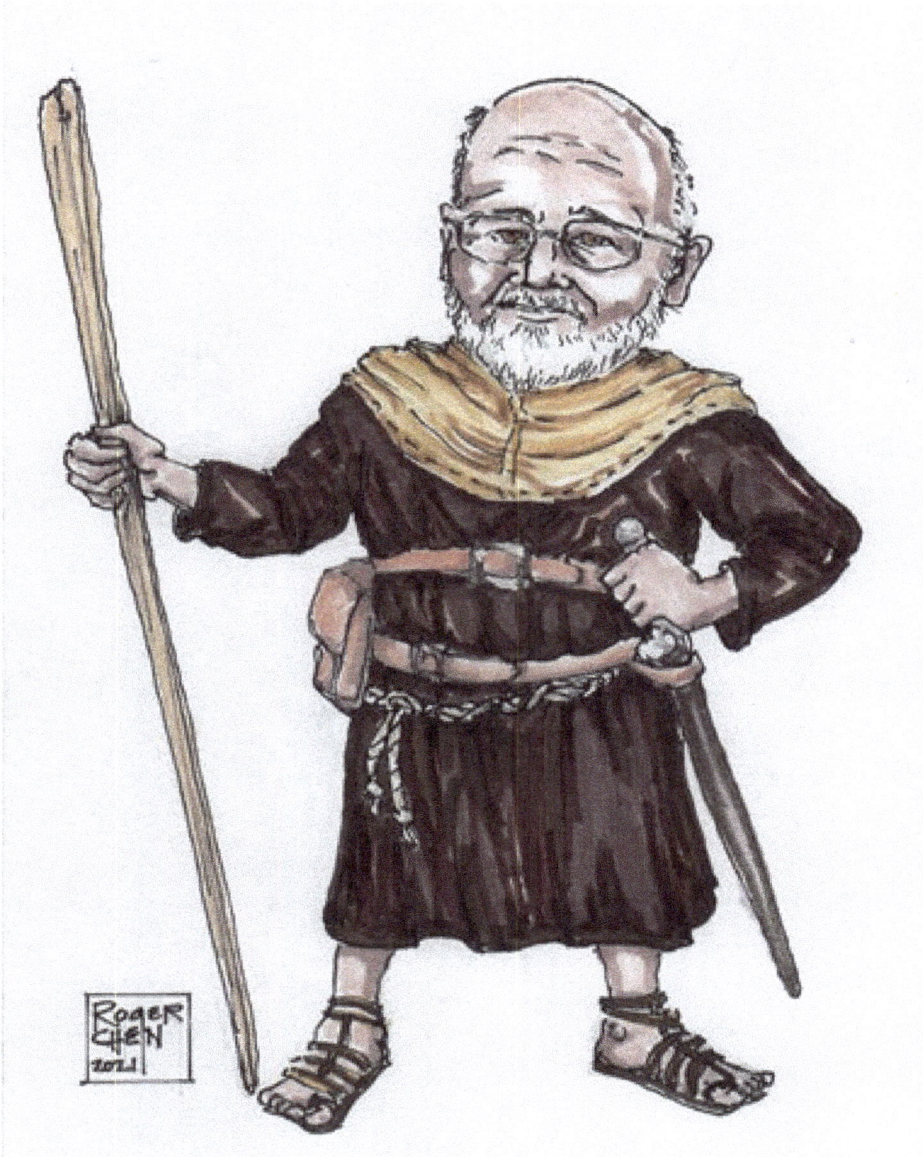

John W. Weisel

John W. Weisel

John Weisel graduated from Swarthmore College in 1968 with a BS in Engineering. He obtained his PhD in 1974 at Brandeis University under the mentorship of *Albert Szent-Györgyi*, a Nobel Laureate (1937). He then spent several years at The Rosenstiel Center at Brandeis University investigating fibrinogen structure with *Carolyn Cohen*. In 1981 he joined the faculty at The University of Pennsylvania in The Department of Cell and Developmental Biology where he has remained to the present.

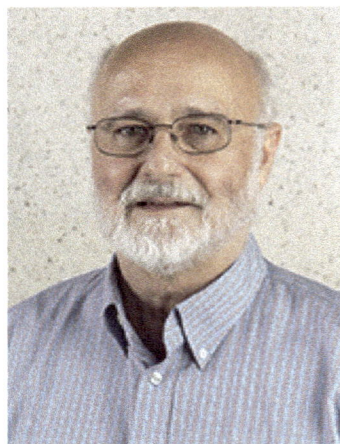

John and I began a letter exchange shortly after his 1993 JBC publication [11], a report that was focused on the location of covalently cross-linked γ chains in fibrin fibrils. Based upon his findings, Weisel concluded that the cross-links were positioned *longitudinally* ('DD-long') between the fibrin molecules that formed each strand of a fibril. His view echoed *Russ Doolittle's* longstanding conjecture and that in Fowler's more recent 1981 report, and ignored Selmayr's two earlier reports (1986, 1988) and one from my group (1989) that provided evidence for a *transverse* cross-linking arrangement, a structure that was morphologically distinct from what they had proposed.

Weisel's report converted what had been a relatively quiescent argument into a more contentious controversy that stimulated several new investigations from my laboratory or that were carried out in collaboration with the STEM group at the Brookhaven National Laboratory. During that same period, Doolittle continued to pursue his 'Holy Grail', which he fervently believed would devolve from his studies of crystallized fibrin D fragments. Other investigators, *Yakovlev and Medved*, reported experiments that led to their *'pullout'* hypothesis that described reversible unfolding of portions of the γ-module in the fibrin(ogen) D Domain. Their discovery effectively neutralized the Doolittle *'distance'* argument that was intended to eliminate the possibility of a *transverse* cross-linking arrangement.

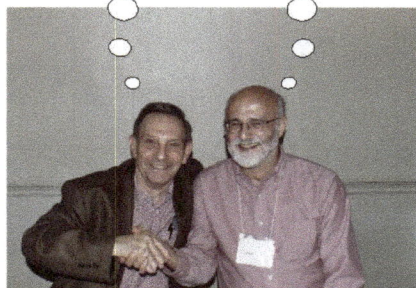

Our letter exchange began in 1993 and continued unabated until 2006. For the most part, these letters were focused on our published reports and vigorous debates concerned with our respective positions in the cross-linking controversy.[6] We also met regularly at different venues to continue our discussions over a lunch or dinner. These communications and meetings were always cordial, never derisive, or dismissive. In retrospect, although John's stubbornness was vexing to me, it was satisfying to have had such an intelligent dialogue with a worthy opponent. We never resolved our differences.

Our meetings and other exchanges lasted until 2006, well beyond publication of our cross-linking 'Debate' articles in 2004. As describing elsewhere, they included plans for a collaborative project that we both agreed could distinguish unambiguously between the two possible cross-linking arrangements. From my standpoint, any new information that we might obtain would likely amount to additional confirmation of existing evidence for a *transverse* cross-linking arrangement. For Weisel, this protocol would have been more perilous, considering the likelihood that the findings would amount to another repudiation of his hypothesis. I was disappointed that the collaboration ended without a resolution.

As described earlier, I paused my involvement in that issue between 2010 to 2020, until coming across *Litvinov* and *Weisel's* 2017 review article entitled '*Fibrin Mechanical Properties and Their Structural Origins*'. This review highlighted the most recent studies on the biophysical properties of fibrin. Almost every study that was cited assumed without attribution, that cross-linked γ chains in fibrin fibrils were aligned *longitudinally*. Not a single article made mention of the controversy that had existed for more than twenty years. The

---

[6] I appended examples of our letter exchanges in Addendums 1 and 2. The ones included concerned Weisel's 1993 JBC publication [11].

Litvinov/Weisel article had reawakened my interest and led shortly afterward to this present narrative.

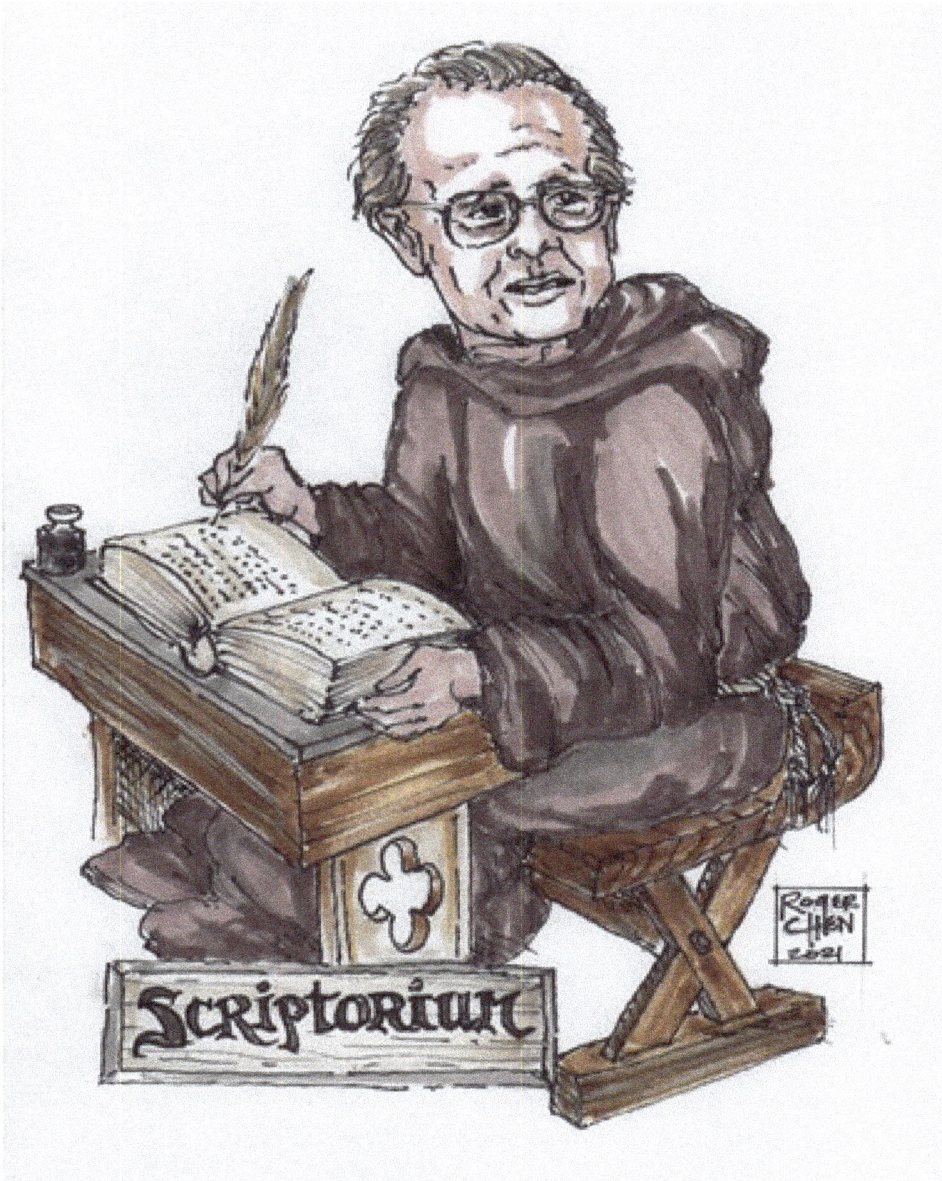

Chapter 7

Laszlo Lorand

Laszlo Lorand

In 1948, *Lazlo Lorand*, a Medical Student at that time, and his mentor, Professor *Koloman Laki* described a new clotting factor in blood that they first named the *Laki-Lorand* Factor. A few years later the 'L-L' Factor, aka *Plasma Transglutaminase*, became widely known as *Factor XIII*. Lorand studied this enzyme, which introduces covalent bonds into fibrin(ogen) and other substrates, for his entire scientific career. When it came to the fibrin cross-linking issue, he also participated.

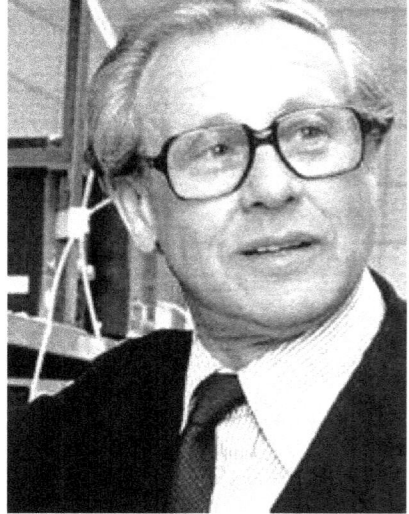

Laci ('Latzi') and I maintained our friendship for nearly fifty years beginning in the 60's at venues ranging from summers at The Marine Biological Laboratory (MBL) at Woods Hole, Massachusetts, Gordon Conferences, and other scientific meetings in numerous locations, including as an invited lecturer at the 2001 New York Academy of Sciences International Symposium on Fibrinogen and at the Blood Research Institute of the BloodCenter of Wisconsin, to 'backyard neighbors' traveling between our homes in Evanston, Illinois and in Milwaukee, Wisconsin. Because of his long ranging involvement in Factor XIII, transglutamination, and the cross-linking issue, I will relate some relevant events in his life and scientific career.

I can attest to or document most events in this narrative myself, or they were transmitted from reliable sources. The narrative reveals Lorand's affable personality, his intelligence, morality, and occasional unethical behavior. I tried not to be judgmental or prescriptive in relating these stories, preferring instead to leave those decisions to readers. In general, the story concerns a skilled and highly competent academic scientist whose legacy was tarnished by accusations of unethical behavior and impropriety bordering on plagiarism.

Lazlo Lorand was born and grew up in Hungary. As alluded to above, in 1948 he and Professor Koloman Laki discovered a serum clotting

28

factor they named the '*Laki-Lorand*' Factor.[7] That same year, during the Cold War, he left Budapest for the University of Leeds where he earned a PhD in Biomolecular Structure (1951). He then immigrated to the United States, joined the faculty at Wayne State University, and subsequently moved to Northwestern University where he spent many years in the Departments of Chemistry and Molecular Biosciences.

During his career he was a productive, knowledgeable, and influential investigator, an impressive and flamboyant speaker with a pleasing British/Hungarian accent and an engaging smile for those upon whom he conferred it (I was one of the lucky ones.). His scientific accomplishments and contributions, especially in elucidating Factor XIII structure and function, were recognized by his election to the National Academy of Sciences.

Doolittle's Complaint

His notable qualities and achievements notwithstanding, Lorand occasionally displayed self-aggrandizing behavior that tarnished his reputation and his scientific legacy. One such episode involved *Russ Doolittle* in 1969: I first became aware that there was an issue between them after I received a copy of a memo from Doolittle that he had distributed to many of his colleagues ['*Addendum 3*']. What follows is the gist of the memo: In April 1969, Doolittle submitted a manuscript for publication in PNAS that included identification of the polypeptide chains in fibrin that were involved in Factor XIII-mediated cross-linking. It contained three new findings: "*1) the 'acceptor sites' in fibrin are on gamma (γ) chains; 2) there are two different types of cross-linked chains, gamma-gamma (γ-γ) and gamma-alpha (γ-α); 3) fibrin beta (β) chains are not involved this process.*" Shortly after it had been accepted for publication, Doolittle sent

---

[7] Laszlo told me that he was a 'Holocaust survivor' who had lived in Hungary during the Nazi occupation and eventually emigrated to the United States. In one story that took place in 1971 at meeting of the New York Academy of Sciences, both Koloman Laki and Lorand were scheduled speakers. *John Finlayson* was the designated session chairperson: There had been some friction between them, likely concerning whether the clotting factor they had discovered jointly should have been called the '**Lorand**-Laki Factor' instead of its original name, the '**Laki**-Lorand Factor'. Before the session began, Laki told Finlayson, "*No fireworks; I'm declaring peace with Lorand.*" When Lorand's turn to speak came he said, unexpectedly and deferentially, "*I am grateful to Dr. Laki, not only for the professional opportunity he offered me, but also for my physical survival.*"

preprints to several colleagues, including Lorand. Within a few days Doolittle received a letter from Lorand pointing out that his group had previously '*reported*' (as a footnote in a 1966 article) that acceptor sites in fibrin were on the gamma chains, and that incorporation of dansyl cadaverine was on those chains. Doolittle deferred to Lorand's assertion and added a statement to his publication citing Lorand's "*unpublished observations*". A few days later Doolittle learned that *Lorand and Chenoweth* were 'reporting their observations' on the incorporation of dansyl cadaverine into fibrin in an article that was communicated to PNAS in May or June 1969 and published in August of that year. A second article authored by *Lorand, Chenoweth and Domanik* that was submitted to 'BBRC' in August 1969, described the same results that Doolittle had reported, including their "*discovery*" of cross-linked γ-α chains, a covalent linkage that he reportedly '*copied*' from Doolittle's original publication, a cross-link between γ and α chains that was eventually shown *not* to exist. There was no coherent explanation for this aberrant behavior.

Doolittle and Lorand had previously spent some time together. After Russ received his Ph D (1961), he worked with Lazlo on the lobster (*Homarus americanus*) clotting system at The Marine Biological Laboratory in Woods Hole, Massachusetts.[8] Following that stint, he relocated to The Karolinska Institute to work with Birger Blombäck on the evolution of vertebrate *Fibrinopeptides*, a subject that subsequently occupied much of his lifelong efforts.

In 1982, Russ and I organized and edited a New York Academy of Sciences Conference entitled: *The Molecular Biology of Fibrinogen*. Lorand was an invited speaker. Following the meeting and before publication of its proceedings, he wrote to me about his concern that Doolittle's response to a question about lobster clotting, had been misrepresented to Lorand's detriment. He wanted assurance that those comments would not be published unedited in the conference proceedings. I telephoned to assure him that those comments would not be published. Lorand's acerbic tone in his response suggested that there previously had been some *bad blood* between them ['*Addendum 4*']. I learned nothing more about his issue with Doolittle.

---

[8] To my knowledge, Lorand and Doolittle had one joint publication [*A New Class of Blood Coagulation Inhibitors*. Lorand L, Doolittle RF, Konishi K, Riggs SK., Arch Biochem Biophys 102:170-179, 1963.]

John Pisano versus Lazlo Lorand

John Pisano, John Finlayson, and *Marjorie Peyton* at The National Institutes of Health (NIH) analyzed an enzymatic hydrolysate of cross-linked fibrin and found conclusive evidence that an ε–(γ–glutamyl) lysine isopeptide bond had been introduced into fibrin. The existence of such a bond in fibrin had been postulated before, but proof had been lacking until their report appeared in 1968.

Their manuscript was submitted to '*Science* on January 19, 1968. In their transmission letter, *John Pisano* requested that because of previous 'conflicting reports', their manuscript should not be sent to *Lazlo Lorand* for review, but any other reviewers were acceptable.[9] Despite Pisano's reservations, the manuscript was sent to Lorand *"forthwith"*. According to Finlayson, *"He sat on it for months."*

Eventually, their paper was published in May 1968. *"During that interval Lorand published our results three times"* wrote Finlayson, *"once was in an addendum to a paper in Biochemistry (March 1968) that was at best, tangentially related to the subject."* Another account appeared in February 1968 in the introduction to a paper in The Journal of Clinical Investigation. Lorand stipulated that fibrin monomers *"cross-link in a transpeptidation reaction to form gamma-glutamyl-epsilon-lysine bonds"*. He supported his statement by citing three publications of his that had appeared in 1966, several years before Pisano's discovery of the ε–(γ–glutamyl) lysine bond.

The third account appeared in the April 1968 issue of Biophysical and Biochemical Research Communications (BBRC). *John Pisano* reportedly commented, *"there was no possible way that the experiment(s) Lorand described in that paper could have yielded the elution pattern that was shown as a figure."*

It is worth noting that even before Lorand's April 1968 communication, *Matiçic* and *Loewy* reported the same results as had Pisano et al. Ironically, their account had been submitted one day before Pisano's on January 18, 1968. Loewy's report was not unexpected since Pisano had taught his colleague, *Ariel Loewy,* the methodology for detecting ε–(γ–glutamyl) lysine, underscoring the collegiality that existed

---

[9] I was aware of their conflictual relationship, having been at a conference session where I heard a vituperative exchange between an angry Pisano and a composed but defensive Lorand. To supplement my knowledge of their dispute, I reached out to John Finlayson to help put a finer point on the details ['*Addendum 5*].

between them.

Robert Bruner and Serendipity

Lazlo Lorand and *Joyce Bruner* met in 1953 and were married in 1955. They eventually settled in the Chicago area at Northwestern University. Joyce was a PhD scientist who retained her maiden name as *Bruner*-Lorand. She worked for many years in her husband's laboratory, and they were co-authors on numerous publications.

In October 1981, a few months after I had moved to Milwaukee to serve two academic roles: Director of The Research Division and Vice Chairman of the Department of Medicine. In the latter capacity, I was serving as an Attending Physician on the Medical Service at Sinai Samaritan Hospital. A patient named *Robert Bruner* was admitted to our Service because of failing health, malnutrition, debilitation, and an inability to care for himself. At the outset of his hospitalization, he was coherent and communicative. I noted immediately that his surname was the same as Joyce *Bruner*-Lorand's. During the admission interview, I asked him whether he had any relatives living in the Midwest. He responded that he had a daughter named Joyce who lived in Chicago, she was married to a scientist, and that they had a daughter named Michele.

Mr. Bruner also said that years before he had left Joyce's home unannounced at about the time, he and Joyce's mother were divorcing. Since his departure he had not contacted her or anyone else in the family. Nevertheless, he resettled near to where they lived and regularly tracked Joyce's whereabouts and her life's activities. I inferred that *Joyce Bruner-Lorand* was *Robert Bruner's* daughter and I telephoned Laci to inform him of my finding. He confirmed that no one in their family had any idea that Robert was still alive and living nearby.

Shortly after that call, Laci drove up to Milwaukee and verified my speculation that Robert was 'Joyce's father', first by speaking with him at length and shortly after that, by visiting Robert's apartment. There he discovered several important documents, including pictures of Joyce and the divorce papers from Joyce's mother, clearly verifying their filial relationship.

In a follow up letter to me the next month ['*Addendum 6*'] Laci revealed that Robert Bruner had served in both World Wars and had received a 30% disability pension at discharge. He wrote poetry and was an expert in American history. Robert died a few days after we had admitted him. His autopsy revealed an underlying metastatic prostate cancer.

Joyce and Michele, their daughter, visited Robert two days after Laci had met with him. Although he was semi-comatose by then, they both felt that he was aware of their presence. Laci told me in a personal conversation sometime after their visit that Joyce and her father had had a close and affectionate relationship and she was grateful to me for having enabled a brief reunion between them before his death. She sent me a note thanking me for that opportunity (*'Addendum 7'*).

Laszlo and Me

Laci and I met in the mid 1960's, a subject I have already touched on. We had numerous meetings over the next 35 years, and despite everything that had happened between him and *Russ Doolittle*, *John Pisano* and others, our own relationship developed as a friendship that did not require trust on my part for it to survive. Despite the converging nature of our own investigations, I had little concern that any of our interactions might engender the subterfuge that he had previously engaged in. I also believed that his prior unseemly behavior belied his worth as an investigator and scientist. Our personal encounters were always cordial and non-confrontational. I last saw him and Joyce in 2010 on a visit to their home in Evanston, Illinois a few days before her death from metastatic ovarian carcinoma.

A few months before that final visit we had had several email exchanges largely concerning our report that a significant portion of the most potent circulating inhibitor of fibrinolysis, α2-antiplasmin, was tightly (covalently) bound to fibrinogen). I devoted an entire chapter to that subject in *Fibrinogen Memoirs* [Chapter IX, *'Addendum 8'*]. Lorand questioned the evidence that I had published for the existence of a covalent linkage between α2-antiplasmin and fibrinogen, a finding strongly implying that circulating Factor XIII was responsible for its presence. [also see *Addendum 9*]

My reports conflicted with Lorand's belief that Factor XIII was an *inactive enzyme precursor* until it was cleaved by thrombin and became the active transglutaminase, Factor XIIIa. The discovery of fibrinogen-bound α2-antiplasmin suggested that this intimate association between inhibitor and substrate plays an important role in regulating the lysis rate of intravascular blood clots. It also inferred that the covalent bonds had been incorporated by circulating Factor XIII. It's not clear whether anything I wrote to him or said changed his thinking on this subject.

For my own part there was never an issue of plagiarism of any aspect of my own published or unpublished work, which I fearlessly shared freely with him. I believe that this was so because my areas of interest did not intrude on the subjects he had previously staked out as his alone and about which he was well informed. Our relationship was always cordial, respectful, and sometimes collaborative.[10] Aspects of his research that were his own conception were well designed, well reported, generally of high quality, and credible, even though not all of them stood the test of re-examination. I still do not understand why such a gifted man ever felt the need to co-opt the work of others when his own contributions were so valuable and meritorious.

---

[10] On one occasion (2001), well before the *Mosesson v Weisel* Debate articles had been conceived (2004), Lazlo asked me to provide him with one of my published diagrams that illustrated the structure of an assembled fibrin fibril and the possible γ chain cross-linking arrangements [*Ann NY Acad Sci* 936:11-30, 2001]. He wanted me to 'adapt' the diagram for a forthcoming *"review on transglutaminases"*. I was happy to comply with that request since my diagram prominently displayed the '*transverse*' arrangement that I had been pushing since the Selmayr's report in 1985. Although he did not agree with me on the cross-linking issue, he nevertheless published the exculpatory diagram that I had given him!

Chapter 8

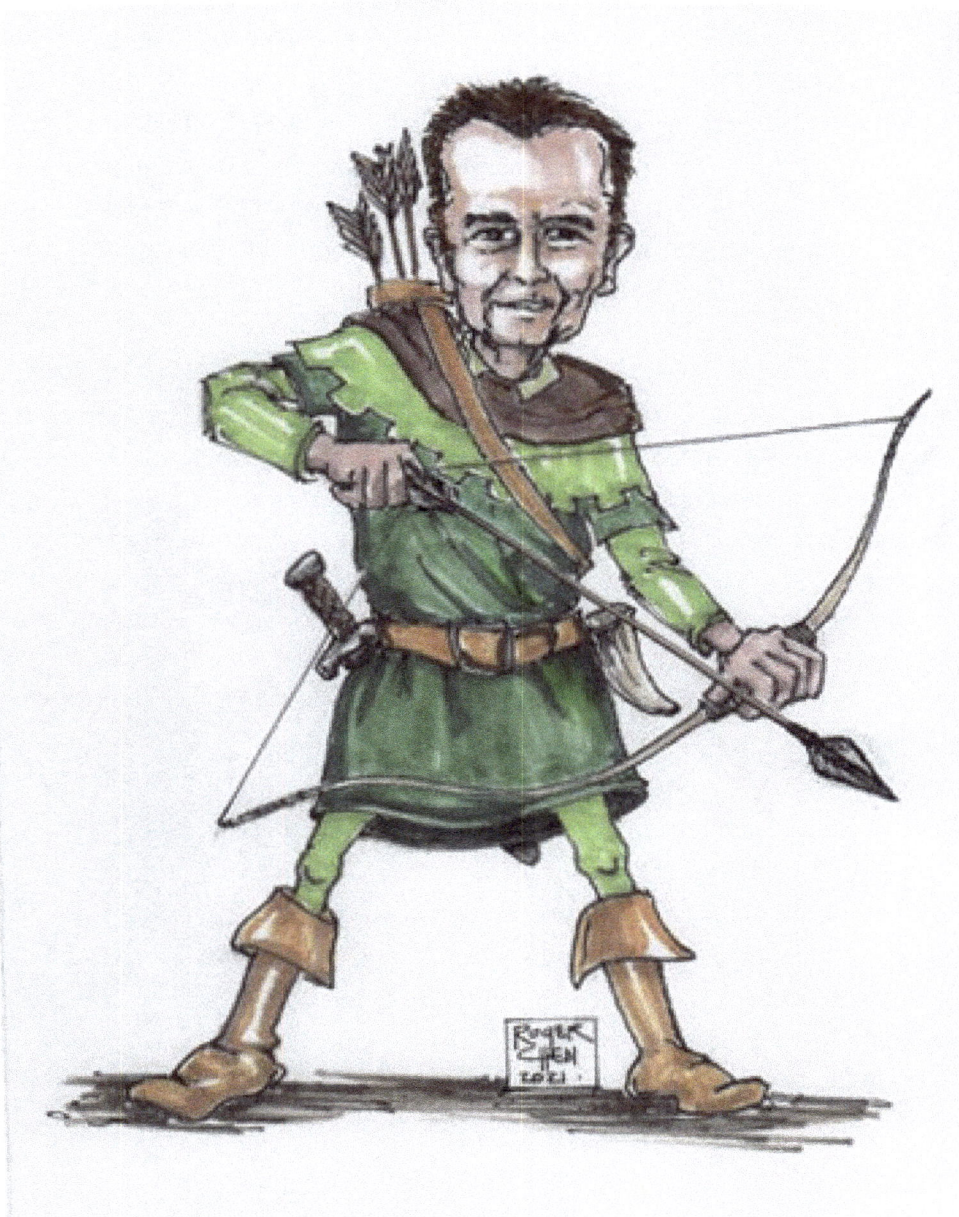

Eberhard Selmayr

Beginnings of the Controversy

The main participants in the controversy that developed were *Eberhard Selmayr, Russ Doolittle, John Weisel, Lazlo Lorand, Leonid Medved, John Ferry,* and me. Until the 1980's there was no experimental evidence for any particular cross-linked γ chain arrangement, though *Russ Doolittle*, as far back as 1973 [6], depicted carboxy-terminal regions of γ chains as squiggly protrusions from the ends of D domains, that interacted with neighboring γ chains in an end-to-end alignment. He perpetuated that fairy tale although concrete evidence for such an arrangment was 'slim to none', then or now.

That was how matters stood until 1981 when *Walter Fowler* published electron micrographs of D-dimers that he found in proteolytic digests of cross-linked fibrinogen [7]. Images of the covalently linked D fragments were aligned *end-to-end* in a so-called 'D-D long' alignment. Fowler reasoned from this observation that it mirrored the intermolecular D Domain arrangement in assembled fibrin fibrils. Although I was aware of that report, I had developed no opinion at that time relating to its veracity or its potential relevance.

About one year later, I accepted an invitation from *Gert Müller Berghaus* to serve on his Scientific Advisory Committee ('Fachbeirat') at Justus-Liebig Universität in Giessen, Germany. At one of the annual visits (1984), I met *Eberhard Selmayr* [11] (*right*) who was in Berghaus' Department as a 'Research Fellow' in partial fulfillment of requirements for his Veterinary Doctor's degree.

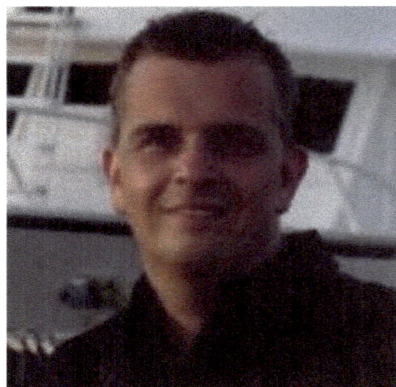

[11] I found a photograph, in an internet search, that I believe to be of *Eberhard Selmayr* taken at about the time he was at Justus-Liebig Universität.

Selmayr was investigating where the carboxy-terminal regions of cross-linked γ chains were positioned in an assembled fibrin clot. I was not aware that an issue existed until he presented his findings at an Advisory Committee meeting. His protocols were designed to distinguish between two possible intermolecular locations, that is, *transverse* or *'DD-long'*. In the experiment illustrated in Figure 3, *fibrin* that had been covalently linked to Sepharose beads was then incubated with *fibrinogen*, followed by Factor XIII addition to produce cross-linking.

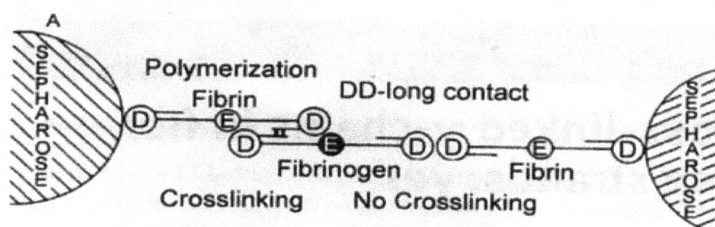

Figure 3. *Selmayr's drawing showing how Sepharose-bound Fibrin would interact with Fibrinogen in the presence of Factor XIII, depending on the orientation of their γ chains. Reproduced from his 1985 publication [8].*

Selmayr reasoned that D Domains of fibrinogen molecules would form non-covalent 'D:E' contacts with the E Domains of the bead-bound fibrin. If the γ chains of the interacting molecules were positioned *'transversely'* between the fibrin and fibrinogen molecules they would become cross-linked, as illustrated on the *left half* of the drawing. If instead, γ chains were positioned in a *'DD-Long'* arrangement (*right half*), cross-linking of fibrinogen to the fibrin-beads would *not* occur or would be greatly reduced compared with *transversely* positioned molecules.

The control arm (not shown) in which bead-bound *fibrinogen* and unbound *fibrinogen* retained their Fibrinopeptides, formed fewer γ chain cross-links than were found in the *fibrin/fibrinogen* experiment (Figure 2). These results demonstrated the importance of D:E contacts for positioning fibrin molecules for 'transverse' ligation. That was a nihilistic proposal at the time, at odds with Fowler's 'D-D long' arrangement. I returned home from the Giessen meeting naïvely believing that once Selmayr's seminal report was published, it would not be long before other investigators reconsidered their views of the fibrin cross-linking arrangement.

Shortly after that groundbreaking first report, Selmayr and I began a collaboration on a project that we hoped would result in imaging the fibrin(ogen) molecules that had been bound to or assembled on Sepharose beads. Although we did succeed in that effort, the findings contributed no new insights into the inquiry, and we did not publish the results. Three years after his first publication, Selmayr published another report on the ultrastructure of urea-dissociated cross-linked fibrin clots [9] which further substantiated earlier conclusions. I urged him to continue his studies, but he had other ideas and soon disappeared into veterinary practice.

As a result of his departure, I decided to join what soon became a full-fledged argument about the arrangement of cross-linked γ chains in fibrin. Doolittle continued to argue against Selmayr's results without offering a sustainable rationale for his beliefs.

I realized that a controversy had arrived. With the help of my associates *Kevin Siebenlist* and *Jim DiOrio*, we began to design experiments that critically examined Selmayr's conclusions. In 1989, we published a report on time-dependent evolution of multimeric cross-linked D fragments in plasmic digests of cross-linked fibrin [10]. In addition to the expected appearance of 'D dimers', we observed time-dependent evolution of higher ordered cross-linked D fragments (i.e., D trimers, D tetramers), findings that were consistent with a *'transverse'* cross-linking arrangement. We were encouraged by these results and continued the quest for more evidence.

Four years after our report, in a work aimed at refuting or nullifying Selmayr's conclusions, *John Weisel* & company fired their opening salvo [11]. They reported their findings on the ultra-structure of cross-linked fragments that had been produced in a proteolytic digest of cross-linked fibrin. Following the digestion phase, they processed specimens in dilute acetic acid, a solution that dissociates non-covalent bonds such as those between D and E Domains (D:E).[12] They then imaged

---

[12] Weisel et al. persisted in disregarding the critical role that *non-covalent* D:E bonding plays in organizing the assembly of fibrin molecules to form double-stranded fibrils. D:E

these digest fragments by transmission electron microscopy (TEM). Under their solvent conditions they found unbound E Domains and cross-linked '*D dimers*' that were aligned end-to-end. These observations were the same as the ones that had been described by Fowler. Weisel mistakenly took this observation as proof for a 'longitudinal' cross-linking arrangement, as illustrated in Figure 4. He ignored Selmayr's earlier reports in framing his arguments and discussion, an unanticipated forerunner of what was to come.

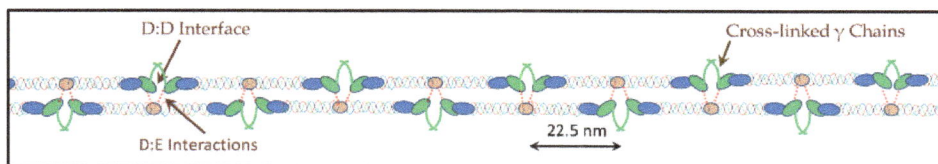

Figure 4. *Drawing of a two-stranded fibril with the cross-linked γ chains* ∧ *positioned between the molecules forming each fibril strand, i.e., 'longitudinally'. Notations are the same as in Figure 1.*

After reading the Weisel paper, we undertook an investigation using STEM imaging of *D-fibrin-D* complexes First, we proved the identity of these complexes by Mass Analysis (see *Addendum 10).* We then evaluated the consequences of applying specimens to a microscope grid under different solvent condition [12]. Specimens that had been applied in a neutral pH saline buffer, showed *D-fibrin-D* complexes that were 'folded' with their outer D Domains situated close to the central E Domain ⬛⬛⬛ of the fibrin molecule, as would be expected when non-covalent D:E interactions are operative. It was also evident that cross-linked γ chains connecting the D Domains in the 'folded' configuration were positioned *transversely*!

When specimens were deposited in an acetic acid solution, *D-fibrin-D* complexes were 'unfolded' and extended ⬛⬛⬛⬛⬛ in a linear configuration, apparently because non-covalent D:E interactions

associations are disrupted in the presence of low pH solutions, such as acetic acid, that they employed in processing their covalently cross-linked specimens for imaging. Dissociation of these bonds disrupts the double-stranded arrangement, which then becomes single-stranded. That occurrence makes it impossible to determine what the arrangement of ligated γ chains had been in the previous double-stranded structure. The same reasoning holds for the covalently cross-linked D dimers in a digest that become dissociated from E fragments for the same reason. We examined that important issue in a set of experiments focused on *cross-linked D-fibrin-D* complexes [12], as described above.

had been disrupted. The configuration of the cross-linked D Domains in D-fibrin-D complexes resembled the 'DD-long' configuration that Fowler and Weisel's had described for cross-linked D-dimers. Our report would be an artful and timely refutation of Weisel's faulty reasoning in the 1993 report. Perhaps it would even end the debate. No such luck–the controversy was just getting underway.

Chapter 9

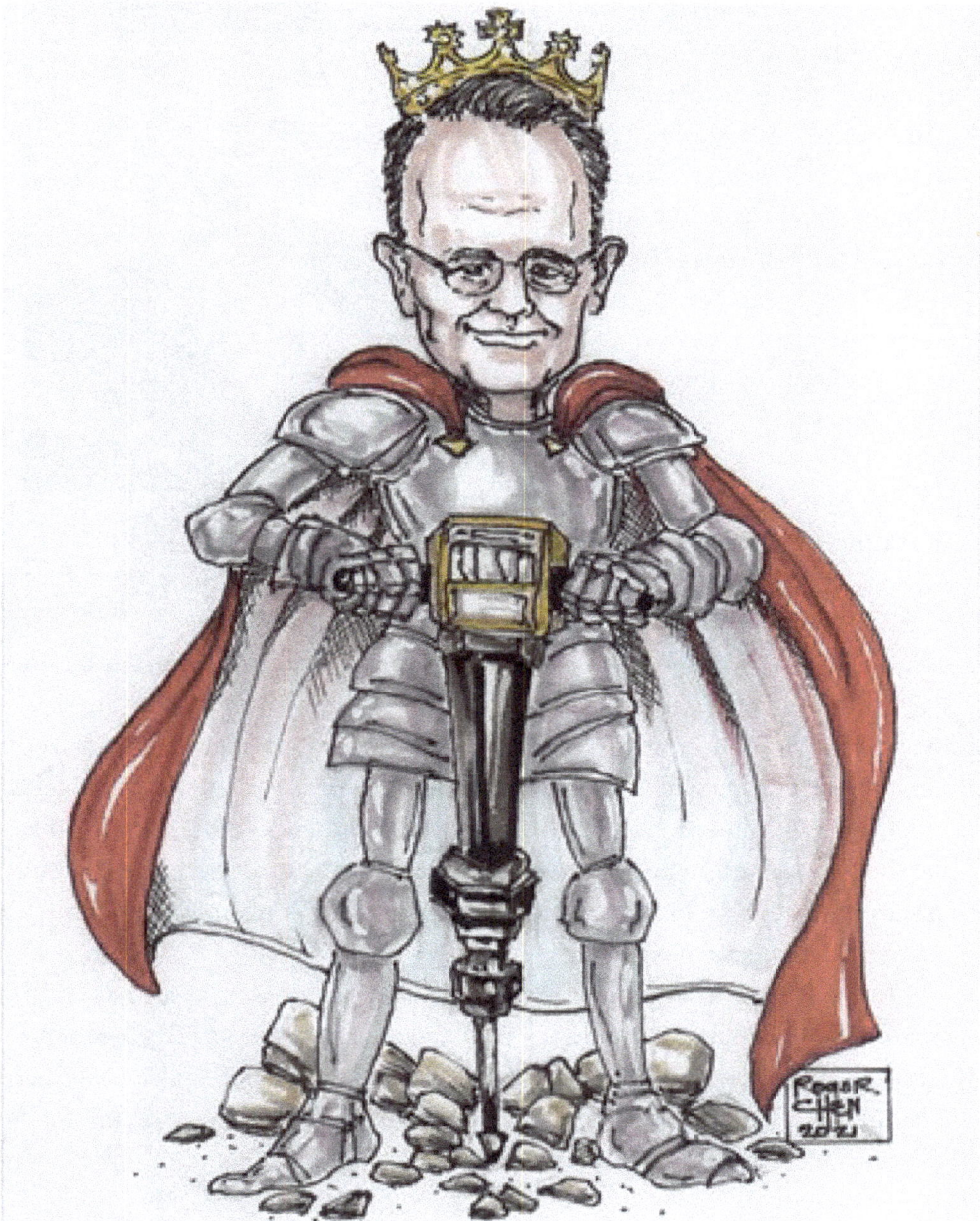

John D. Ferry

John Douglass Ferry

I met John Ferry shortly after relocating from New York to The Milwaukee Clinical Campus of The University of Wisconsin Medical School at Sinai Samaritan Hospital in Milwaukee. I had moved there to develop a Research Division at The Winter Research Institute where I would conduct research, teaching, and clinical activities for the next eighteen years. I also received a collateral appointment to the faculty of The Department of Medicine at The University of Wisconsin in Madison where *John Ferry*, a living legend by that time, was the retired Chairman of The Department of Chemistry on the Madison campus, who was still

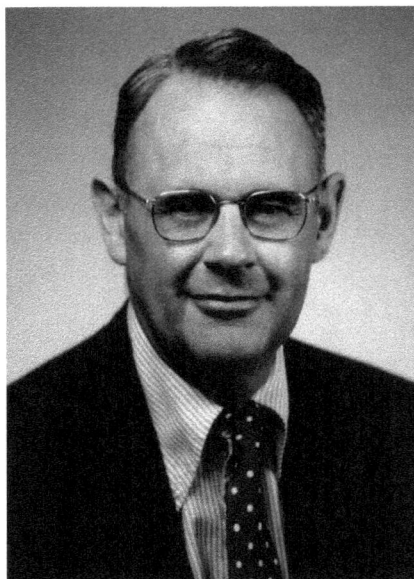

1912-2002

ensconced in his office and actively engaged in research activities as the Farrington Daniels Research Professor (1973). He was an icon in the field of polymer science. His work on Fibrinogen and its polymerized derivative, Fibrin, was familiar to me long before we met. At our first meeting in 1981 he proved to be everything I had earlier imagined him to be, thoughtful, interactive, knowledgeable, and as humble and deferential as he was wise. Informal meetings with him and my group became a regular occurrence over the next fifteen years.

In 1982, I invited him to be the Keynote Speaker at a New York Academy of Sciences conference on *Molecular Biology of Fibrinogen and Fibrin*. [*The Conversion of Fibrinogen to Fibrin. Events and Recollections from 1942 to 1982*. Ferry, JD in *Ann NY Acad Sci*. Vol. 408 (Mosesson, MW and

Doolittle, RF, eds.) p. 1-10, 1983.] His dynamic presentation[13] was the highlight of the meeting that remains fresh in my mind. A few years later when he was closing his laboratory, he graciously offered to transfer his many-meters-long 'homemade' optical bench to my laboratory. I declined, knowing that I lacked the know how to reconstruct, let alone utilize, such a device.

Robert F. Landel, John L Schrag and I memorialized Ferry's life and scientific career in a chapter written for the National Academy of Sciences [*Biographical Memoirs.* Landel RF, Mosesson MW, Schrag JL. *Natl Acad Sci (USA)* 90:86-111, 2009.]. There have been numerous other tributes to his accomplishments, including a *Festschrift* in his honor that I edited with *Enrico Di Cera* [*John D Ferry-Special Issue* [Mosesson MW and Di Cera E, Eds.) *Biophys* J 112:89-302, 2004].

John Ferry was born in Dawson, the Yukon Territory of Canada. His father was a civil and mining engineer specializing in prospecting for placer deposits (panning for gold), a skill he learned and reportedly retained throughout his lifetime. His childhood was spent in mining communities in Idaho and Oregon where he completed his first eight grades in a one room schoolhouse in only four years. During his High School years, he taught himself enough Latin and German to later enter advanced courses in those subjects; languages remained as a lifelong avocation of his. Ferry attended Stanford University and received an AB degree in 1932. After graduation, he became a research assistant at the Hopkins Marine Station at Stanford University. Following that, he relocated to Harvard University where he subsequently became a Junior Fellow of the Society of Fellows at Harvard, a position that enabled him to pursue studies of his own choice, and those were focused on the viscoelastic properties of polymers. During World War II he was attached

---

[13] Ferry wrote: *"Elastic deformation seems to take place primarily by reversible bending and orientation of the large 'ligated' (my insertion) fiber bundles,....". In stretched unligated films, there is slow relaxation of stress and permanent deformation, probably due to slippage **within** the fiber bundles."* Those observations provided a clear distinction between the elasticity of ligated fibrin films and the inelasticity of non-ligated films. Thanks to Ferry's insightful comments and pencil drawings that he bestowed upon me several years later, we were able to attribute those properties to *transverse* location of ligated γ chains.

to a top-secret project at The Protein Foundation, headed by *EJ Cohn*, whose objective was the development of methods for purification of plasma proteins for clinical use by the armed forces. Plasma Fibrinogen was among them, and thus began a career-long interest in fibrinogen and its conversion to fibrin. In collaboration with *Peter Morrison*, they developed fibrin products that were used during the war, including Fibrin Film and Fibrin Foam.

He joined the faculty of the Department of Chemistry of the University of Wisconsin in 1946, was a founding member of the Rheology Research Center and served as departmental Chairman between 1959 and 1967. Ferry's subsequent interest and devotion to fibrinogen and fibrin resulted in some monumental achievements, including the elucidation of the half-staggered molecular arrangement of fibrin molecules in an assembled fiber. [*The Mechanism of Polymerization of Fibrin. Ferry* JD, *Proc Natl Acad Sci USA* 18:566-9, 1952]. Other studies of the biomechanical properties of fibrin [*Studies of Fibrin Films. I. Stress Relaxation and Birefringence. Roska* FJ, Ferry JD, *Biopolymers* 21:1811-32, 1982; *Studies of Fibrin Films. II. Small-Angle X-Ray Scattering*. Roska FJ, Ferry JD, *Biopolymers* 21:1833-45, 1982] were keys to our understanding of the relationship between the elastic properties of fibrin and the arrangement of cross-linked γ chains in fibrin fibrils.

Although revered for work related to Fibrin, his contributions to polymer science elevated him to the status of Legend. The theme of Ferry's inquiries always revolved around the relationship between molecular motion in macromolecules and their mechanical and other physical properties. The scope of his work included a broad spectrum of systems, ranging from dilute and concentrated solutions to undiluted bulk polymers, both ligated and unligated. His studies of rubbers, polymer melts and solutions provided a foundation in mechanical properties for scientists in industry and academia. His textbook *'Viscoelastic Properties of Polymers'* was first printed in 1961 and was a classic. It was published in two updated editions (1971, 1980) and has been translated into Japanese, Polish, and Russian.

During his career he received many national and international awards. He was elected to membership in the National Academy of

Sciences in 1959. He received the Eli Lilly Award in Biological Chemistry, the Kendall Award in Colloid Chemistry of The American Chemical Society, the High Polymer Physics Prize of the American Physical Society, and the Charles Goodyear Medal of the Rubber Division of the American Chemical Society. His name appears in the Rubber Hall of Fame in Akron, Ohio.

John Ferry was an extraordinary scientist, a dedicated teacher and mentor, admired for his encyclopedic knowledge, his ethics and integrity, his linguistic abilities, and his unparalleled capacity to interpret structural features in terms of the physical properties of a polymer. The last quality was of immeasurable value for our studies of cross-linked fibrin.

Chapter 10

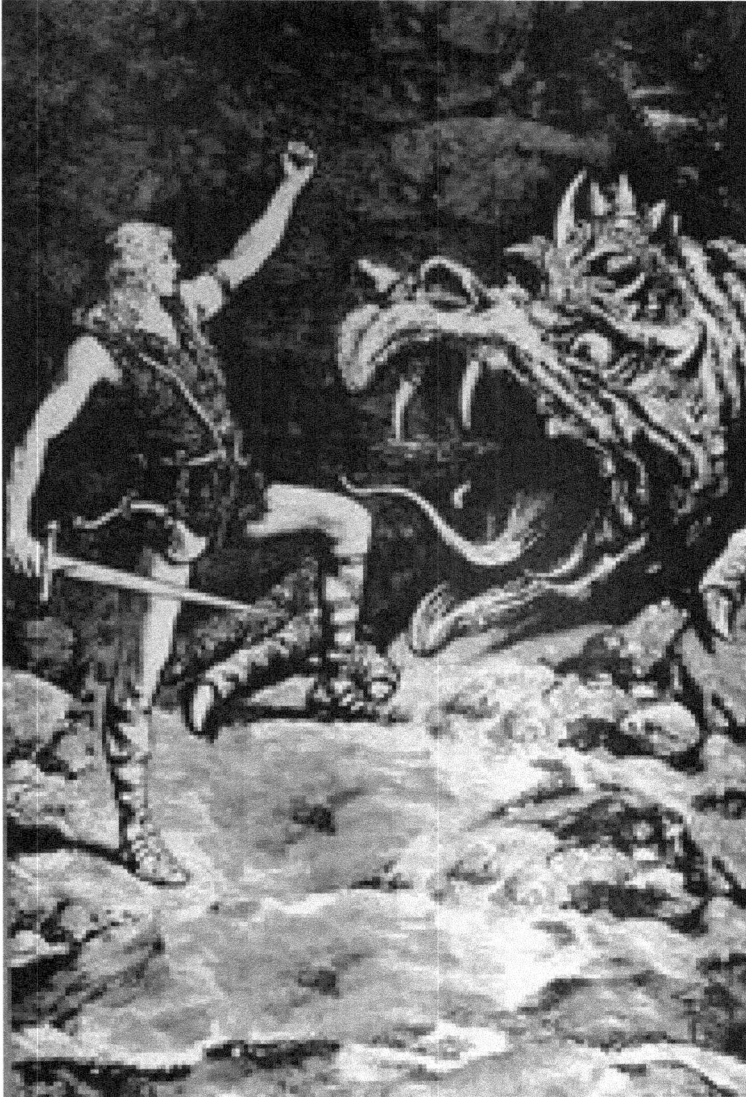

Slaying the Dragon

Transversely Cross-linked Fibrinogen Fibrils

In the experiments described in this chapter, we used thrombin inactivated FXIIIa[14] to produce γ chain cross-linked *fibrinogen*.[15] We then examined specimens by TEM or STEM. The latter technique, which was carried out at The Brookhaven National Laboratory (BNL) STEM facility in collaboration with *Jim Hainfeld* and *Joe Wall*, permitted unambiguous identification of the molecular assemblies and subdomains by determining their mass [13].[16]

It took several weeks of repeatedly studying the STEM images to realize what had occurred. It led to a *Eureka* moment! Cross-linked *fibrinogen* fibrils, similar to fibrin fibrils, had formed half-staggered, double-stranded structures displaying 22.5 nm periodicity as illustrated above and as diagrammed in greater detail in Figure 5. These structures had formed *without* benefit of the non-covalent D:E interactions that drive the assembly of fibrin fibrils. Instead, *fibrinogen fibril* assembly had been driven solely by cross-linking of γ chains that were *transversely* positioned! This, in turn, suggested that the carboxy terminal regions of fibrinogen γ chains, prior to cross-linking,

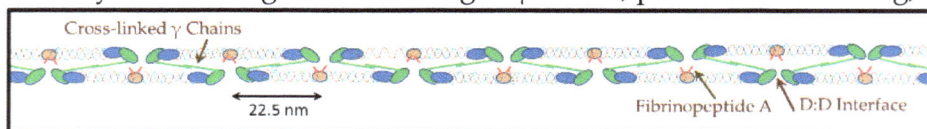

Figure 5. *Drawing of a cross-linked Fibrinogen Fibril. Double-stranded fibrils form because of the transversely positioned cross-linked γ chains. Domains and substructural designations are the same as in Figure 1.*

---

[14] Native plasma Factor XIII (FXIII) possesses nearly as much cross-linking potential for fibrinogen and fibrin as does thrombin activated FXIII (FXIIIa) [14] although the equivalency does not hold for synthetic substrates. When thrombin activity in FXIIIa is inhibited with Hirudin, its activity is equivalent to that of native FXIII and it yields the same cross-linked product with fibrinogen as the substrate. Because of their equivalency in our experiments, I frequently use 'FXIII' to represent either form.

[15] For these experiments we used Des /α Fibrinogen- (i.e., Subfraction I-9) which possesses truncated α chains (α/) that lack cross-linking sites. When this fibrinogen is subjected to cross-linking by FXIII or FXIIIa, only the γ chains become ligated.

[16] *Addendum* 10 contains a description of STEM and Mass Analysis of STEM images, and an account of their invaluable role in nailing down our conclusions.

tend to be oriented toward the center of the molecule, a subject that we would address in detail somewhat later.

In studies of cross-linked *fibrinogen* fibrils, we also examined negatively contrasted specimens by TEM (Figure 6). We found *fibrinogen fibrils* and *multi-stranded fibers* that had formed through lateral associations of its constituent fibrils. The fibers showed 22.5 nm periodicity, demonstrating how closely they resembled *fibrin* fibers. These results, taken together with earlier studies, including Selmayr's reports, bolstered our confidence in positioning cross-linked γ chains in a *transverse* arrangement.

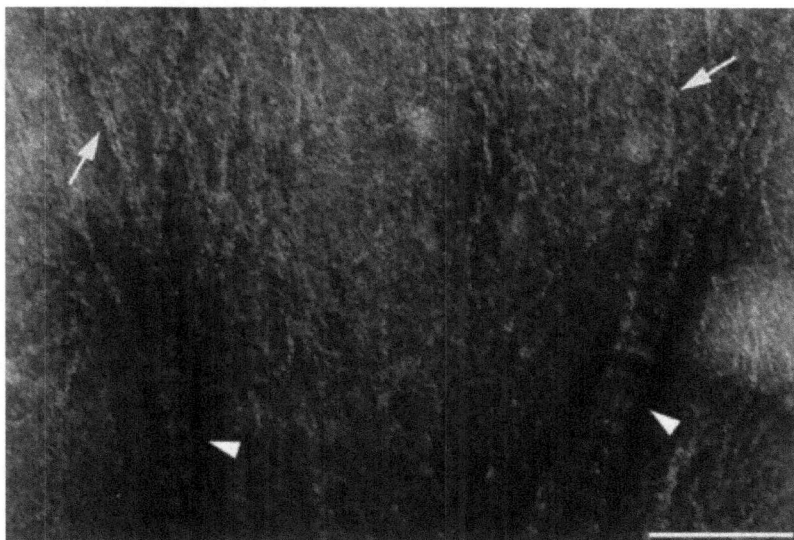

*Figure 6. A TEM image of negatively contrasted cross-linked **fibrinogen** fibrils (arrows) and laterally associated fibrils that had coalesced to form **fibrinogen** fibers (arrowheads). These fibers displayed 22.5 nm periodicity. Bar, 100 nm. Adapted from Ref 13.*

My confidence in these conclusions notwithstanding, I was unable to relate the *transverse* cross-linking arrangement to a known property of a fibrin polymer. *John Ferry,* whose bio-sketch is in the preceding chapter, led me to the solution a few weeks after we had presented our findings to him (1996) at a meeting in a Madison Bed-and-Breakfast Inn dining room. (*photo*). A few days after that memorable occasion, Ferry sent me a letter containing a pencil drawing (Figure 7). In the letter he explained that fourteen years earlier (1982) he and *FJ Roska* had studied the elastic properties of cross-linked fibrin polymers and found them to exhibit perfect *elasticity*. With that simple drawing Ferry had linked his results on cross-linked fibrin elasticity

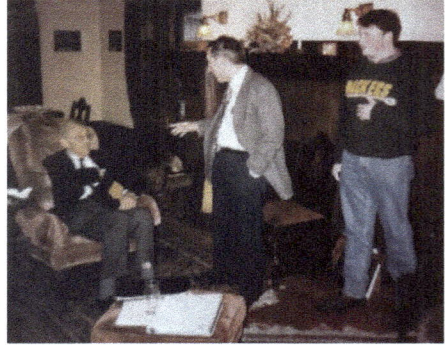

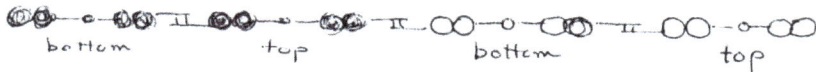

Figure 7. *John Ferry's pencil drawing of a stretched 'single-stranded' cross-linked fibril produced from a double-stranded fibrin fibril. 'Top' and 'Bottom' refer to fibrin molecules derived from opposing transversely cross-linked strands of a fibril. The location of these 'top strand' and 'bottom strand' molecules in an unstretched cross-linked fibril are redrawn below in* **Figure 8**

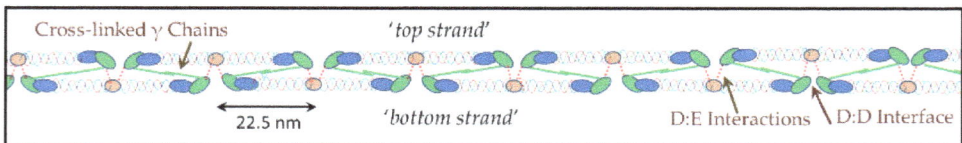

Figure 8. *Figure 4 has been labeled to indicate the* **'top strand'** *and* **'bottom strand'** *molecules in an unstretched fibril.*

to our own results. In a few 'strokes of a pencil' he revealed the connection that I had sought between fibrin's elasticity and *transverse* cross-linking. I was thrilled when I finally grasped those insights.

That revelation led to entitling Chapter VI, '*Fibrin, The Perfect Bioelastomer*', and dedicating the book to *John Ferry's* memory. Beyond that, the observation that γ chain cross-linked *fibrinogen* fibrils formed solely due to *transverse* positioning of cross-linked γ chains, gave me confidence to conclude that at last we had finally '*Slain the Dragon*'. Alas, my conclusion was premature.

Chapter 11

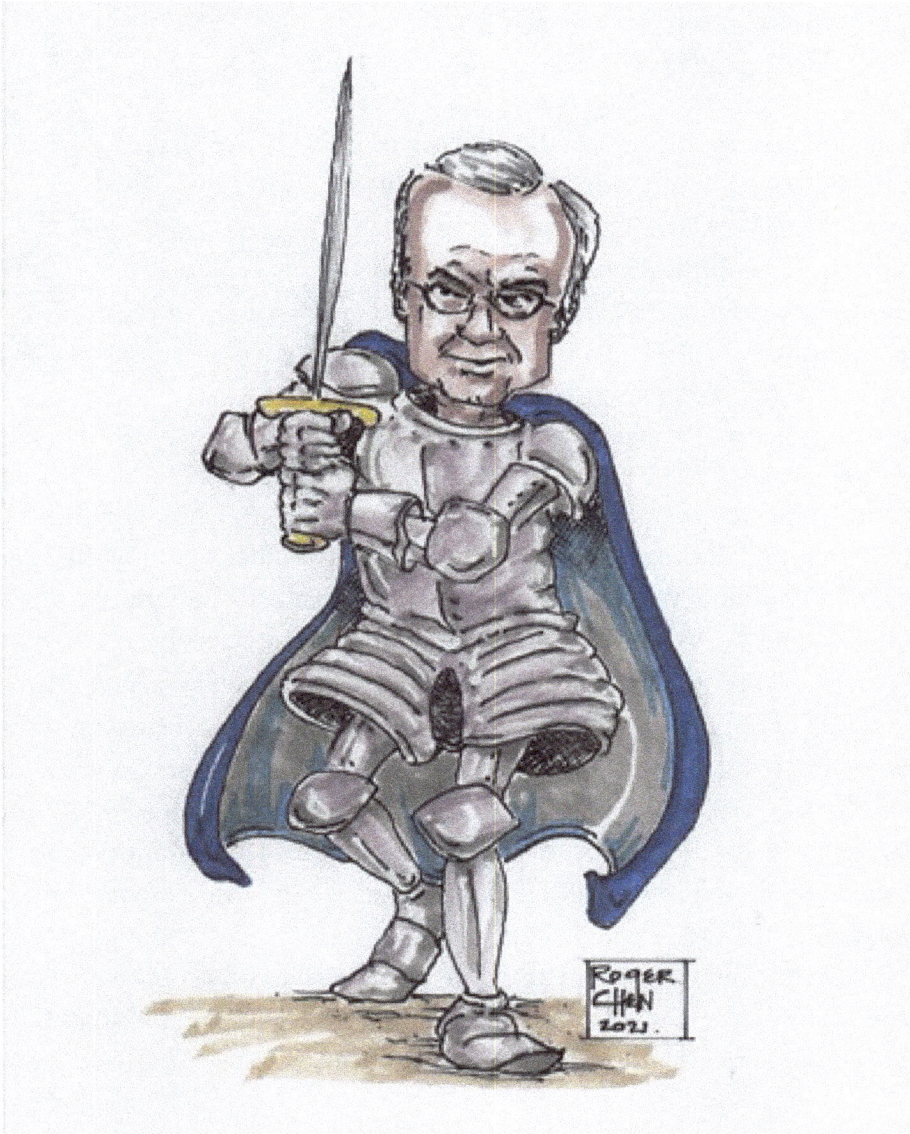

Leonid V. Medved

Leonid V. Medved

*L*eonid Medved was born and educated in Ukraine. He earned a master's degree in Biophysics at Shevchenko University in Kyiv, Ukraine (1977) and a PhD in Biochemistry at The Institute of Biochemistry of The National Academy of Sciences of Ukraine in Kyiv (1980). Between 1981 and 1983 he pursued further training in application of differential scanning calorimetry for analysis of plasma protein structure at The Institute of Protein Research in Pushchino, Russia with Professor *Peter Privalov* and at The Institute of Biochemistry with Professor *Vladimir A. Belitser.* In 1987 he became Head of The Department of Protein Structure and Function at The Institute of Biochemistry in Kyiv, a position he held for ten years. While serving in that capacity, he spent several years as a Visiting Scientist at The J. Holland Laboratory of The American Red Cross in Rockville, Maryland working closely with *Kenneth C. Ingham* [17] in the Biochemistry Department. While working at The Holland Laboratory, he was also teaching at The Department of Biochemistry and Molecular Biology at George Washington University in Washington, DC, where he rose to the rank of Professor between 2000 and 2004. Since 2004 he has been at The University of Maryland School of Medicine in Baltimore, MD, as Professor in the Department of Biochemistry and Molecular Biology.

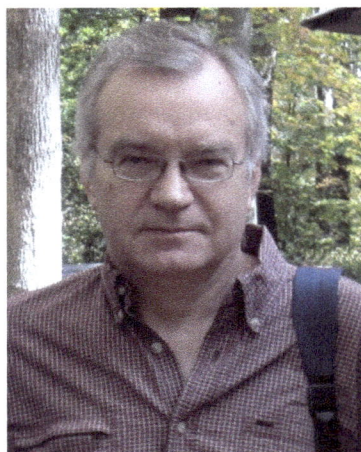

While he was working in Kyiv, he received numerous awards and headed his own Department at The Institute of Biochemistry. Since relocating to the United States, Leonid has been widely recognized for his

---

[17] In Ken's Autobiography [*Feet in the City, Heart on the Farm*. Ingham KC. *Ingham KC, Pub.* (p. 1-434, 2013) ISBN 13-;978-1479110360.] he described his visit to Russia and Ukraine, how difficult it had been (while Ukraine was part of the USSR) to arrange for Leonid to be a Visiting Scientist at the Holland Laboratory. He also wrote about Leonid's excellence as an investigator, and their cordial relationship.

numerous academic, scientific, teaching, and mentoring accomplishments at George Washington University and The University of Maryland School of Medicine. His research activities have been continuously supported by NIH grants since 1998. He was the recipient of a *Fogarty International Research Collaborative Award* (1993), served as President of *The International Fibrinogen Research Society (IFRS)* (2010-2014) and was awarded an *Outstanding Investigator Award* by the IFRS (2000). He was twice an Editor of *Thrombosis Research* (1989-93, 1998-2003) and Section Editor of *Thrombosis and Haemostasis (2006-)*.

I was familiar with Leonid's published work that had originated in Ukraine, but I did not meet him until 1988 at the Fibrinogen Workshop in Milwaukee. From there our relationship and interactions grew rapidly, and led to increased scientific discussions, several collaborative studies, and a close friendship. I was honored to support his candidacy for promotion to *Senior Scientist* at The Holland Laboratory (2000).

Leonid began his research career by studying the domain structure of the fibrinogen molecule using Differential Scanning Calorimetry. He then focused on the structure and function of plasma proteins that are involved in blood coagulation and fibrinolysis.

Subsequently, his interests turned to fibrin(ogen) structure and the molecular mechanisms of its interactions with plasma proteins and cellular receptors. These studies were important for this present narrative because they provided a missing link in the accumulated chain of evidence for a *transverse* cross-linking arrangement. Specifically, his work demonstrated how reversible unfolding of the γ module in the D domain of fibrinogen occurs, resulting in exposure of cryptic cellular binding sites and enabling cross-linking of *transversely* positioned γ chains in fibrin [i, ii]. They were of great value for dissembling *Russ Doolittle's* contention that there was "*not enough distance for a transverse arrangement*" (see Figure below).

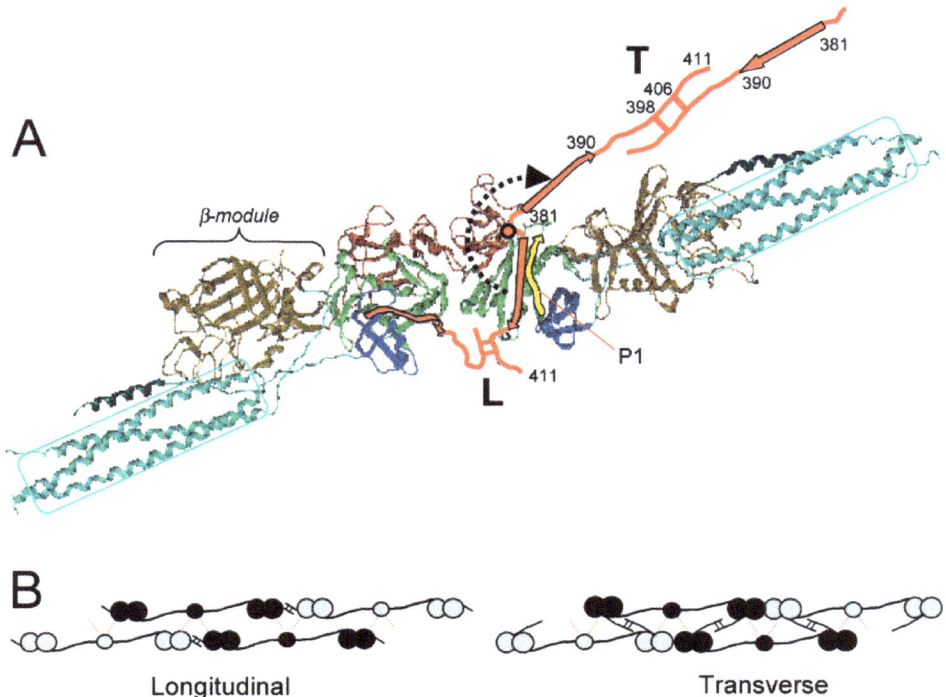

Figure. *The 'pullout' hypothesis explains how transversely positioned, cross-linked γ chains form in fibrin fibrils. Panel **A** illustrates how an embedded 'β-strand insert' (red ribbon with arrowhead) in the central domain of the γ-module (green ribbon) can be pulled out from this domain (The dotted **black** arrow) to enable transverse γ chain cross-linking (**T**). Panel **B** illustrates schematically the longitudinal and transverse arrangements in a fibrin fibril. Reproduced from Ref. i.*

Literature Citations

i.   ROLE OF THE β-STRAND INSERT IN THE CENTRAL DOMAIN OF THE FIBRINOGEN γ-MODULE. Yakovlev S, Litvinovich S, Loukinov D, Medved L. *Biochemistry* 39:15721-29, 2000.

ii. INTERACTION OF FIBRIN(OGEN) WITH LEUKOCYTE RECEPTOR $\alpha_M\beta_2$ (MAC-1): FURTHER CHARACTERIZATION AND IDENTIFICATION OF A NOVEL BINDING REGION WITHIN THE CENTRAL DOMAIN OF THE FIBRINOGEN GAMMA-MODULE. Yakovlev S, Zhang L, Ugarova T, Medved L. *Biochemistry* 44:617-26, 2005.

Chapter 12
More Evidence for a Transverse Arrangement

In 1995, after completing the *Cross-linked Fibrinogen Fibril* project (Ref. 13), I paid a self-styled visit to *Russ Doolittle* to share these findings with him, hoping in vain to persuade him to reconsider his views. Russ was not welcoming, did only a perfunctory examination of information I had brought with me to show him, without offering a single substantive comment. Further details about that visit were recorded in Chapter VI of *Fibrinogen Memoirs* [2].[18]

The following year (1997) Russ published the X-ray structure of crystallized D fragments and cross-linked D-dimers ⬤◖⬤ that he termed *'Double-D'* [15]. Although he could not locate the cross-linked γ chains connecting the D domains in the crystal structure, he inferred that they bridged between them (the dotted segment bridging between D Domains). More problematically, he also inferred from these structures that this location constituted 'proof' that cross-linked γ chains in fibrin were situated *'longitudinally'* along each strand of a fibril.

Three years after our landmark 1995 publication on *'Cross-linked Fibrinogen Fibrils'* [13], *Yuri Veklich* from Weisel's group published results of experiments in which fibrinogen molecules had been assembled on a fibrin Fragment *E* template (*des AB-Fragment E*), and then cross-linked with FXIIIa [16]. Following that phase, they processed the product for imaging in an *acetic acid* solution (just as they had done in their 1993 report) and then examined the product by TEM. Not surprisingly, since

---

[18] This was not the only time Russ had been in an adversarial situation. A few years earlier, he launched a campaign against *Agnes Henschen* who he depicted as *'A Panzer Division'* in an article in a San Diego newspaper that carried the gratuitous heading 'GERMAN RESEARCHERS HOT ON THE TRAIL OF SAME DISCOVERY'. Henschen was a well-regarded Biochemist who used the *'Edman'* amino acid sequencing technique to determine the sequence of fibrinogen. That was a more advanced technique than had previously existed, one she had learned from its inventor, *Per Edman*, her late husband. Accordingly, Doolittle did not win the 'sequencing race' and as told by *Henschen* and *Lottspeich*, he had made errors in the sequence that he reported, a revelation that served to sour their relationship even further.

the non-covalent bonds between the D and E domains had dissociated under their solvent conditions, they found cross-linked single fibril *strands* and unbound E fragments. Based on these findings they once again proffered this as evidence for a *longitudinal* cross-link arrangement in fibrin.

That same year, Lorand et al. [17] published his findings concerning the assembly and cross-linking of D Domains in the presence of a synthesized divalent peptide ligand that was functionally equivalent to a Fibrin E Fragment lacking Fibrinopeptide A (*des A Fragment E).* They analyzed the products of their experiment by gel electrophoresis and found that the addition of the ligand increased cross-linked D dimer formation. They inferred that this finding was evidence for *longitudinal* positioning of cross-linked γ chains in assembled *fibrin* fibrils. (*The same problematic inference drawn by Doolittle and Weisel.)*

Four years later (2002), we published findings that countered the Veklich et al. experiments and inferences [18]. Our protocols differed from theirs in that we used *two* forms of *Fibrin Fragment E* as templates for assembly of fibrinogen molecules. The first lacked Fibrinopeptides A (*des A-Fragment E),* and the second, like Veklich's, lacked Fibrinopeptides A and B (*des AB-Fragment E).* We evaluated both intact Fibrinogen and Fibrinogen lacking the Aα chain FXIII-reactive sites (*des /α Fibrinogen)*[19]. The latter plasma fibrinogen subfraction served to assure that the observed structural assemblies were attributable solely to ligation of γ chains.

Specimens for imaging were processed in non-dissociating *physiological saline* buffers. We avoided using dissociating acetic acid solutions! The results depended upon which form of *Fragment E* we had employed as template. With des *AB-Fragment E,* we observed double- and multi-stranded fibrils plus complex aggregates, findings that were only consistent with a *transverse* cross-linking arrangement.

---

[19] Des /α Fibrinogen (i.e., 'plasma Fraction I-9') lacks the carboxy-terminal regions of Aα chains containing FXIII cross-linking sites (also see footnotes 4, 15, and Figure 1).

More conclusive evidence for a *transverse* arrangement was forthcoming using *des A-Fragment E* as the template for fibril assembly. Under that condition, double-stranded half-staggered fibrinogen fibrils formed that were nearly identical in appearance to those we had previously demonstrated in *cross-linked fibrinogen fibril* experiments [13] (Figure 9). Both assembly conditions point to a *transverse* cross-linking arrangement and leave no other option.

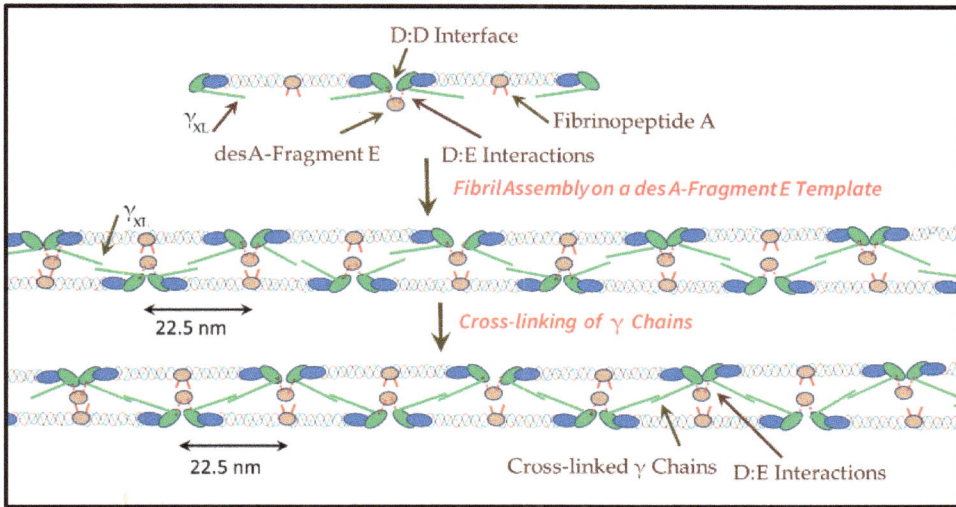

Figure 9. *(**Top row**) Drawing of two fibrinogen molecules that are interacting with **des A Fragment E** ⬤. The fibrinogen E domains retain both FPA and FPB and the carboxy-terminal regions of γ chains ◢ are positioned 'transversely' relative to its parent molecule. (**Middle row**) Fibrinogen molecules assembled on des A-Fragment E-form double- stranded fibrils by virtue of γ chain interactions at γxL sites. (**Bottom row**) The same assembled fibril that has been cross-linked in a 'transverse' arrangement. Its features reflect what we observed by STEM!*

In the same year that *Veklich's* report issued (1998) we published the results of a study designed to locate the carboxy-terminal regions of γ chains in *fibrinogen* molecules and in *fibrin fibrils* [19]. To accomplish this, we employed a lysine amine donor, *cadaverine*,[20] that had been tagged with an electron dense gold cluster [Au_{11},⬤] and readily identifiable by STEM. Using FXIII for transglutamination, we labelled γ chain glutamine

---

[20] The lysine residue in cadaverine replaced the γ406 lysine 'donor' residue that usually participates in cross-linking of γ chains.

acceptor sites in fibrin(ogen) or in fibrin fibrils with Au_{11}-*cadaverine* and then imaged the labelled products using STEM. Under both conditions, we found most of the gold clusters *between the D and E domains* of fibrinogen or fibrin and some were closer to E domains than to D Domains. Most Au_{11} clusters were positioned 'transversely' as if prepared for ligation. These gold clusters would not have been found that far from their origin in the γ module of the D Domain unless some unfolding of the γ-module had occurred.

Studies showing how cross-linked γ chains could become positioned *transversely* between strands of a fibril, were reported about a year later when Yakovlev et al. [20] reported that a '*β-strand insert*' situated within the central domain of the γ-module could unfolded and extend from the module without disrupting overall domain structure (see Figure 10, next page). These findings led to the '*pull out*' hypothesis, namely that unfolding of the '*β-strand insert*' from the central domain of the γ-module permitted contiguous carboxy-terminal regions of the γ chains containing its cross-linking sites to extend far enough between fibril strands, to allow γ chain cross-linking in a *transverse* arrangement.

Russ Doolittle's assertion that there was "*not enough distance for a transverse arrangement*" [21] had been elegantly demolished by this group. Russ nevertheless continued to promote the same dogma, as did Zhmurov et al. [21] [22] in 2016 who used high resolution Atomic Force Microscopy (AFM) to explore the ultrastructure of cross-linked double-stranded fibrin(ogen) oligomers. The investigators were unable to resolve carboxy-terminal portions of the ligated γ chains (γ395-411) that resided within these structures by AFM, yet they inferred that cross-linked γ chains were positioned *longitudinally*. To bolster that unjustifiable speculation, they invoked Doolittle's '*distance*' argument and also remarked that there *had been* a 'Cross-linking Controversy', but that was as far as they ventured in acknowledging that such a controversy still held sway.

---

[21] *Litvinov* and *Weisel* were among the co-authors on that publication, as they had been on most of the related articles published between 2010 and 2020 dealing with biomechanical properties of fibrin.

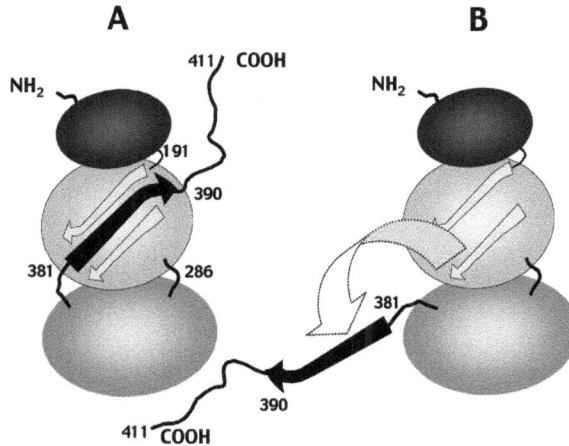

Figure 10. *The 'Pull out' hypothesis explained by this schematic drawing of the γ-module **before**, panel **A**, and **after**, panel **B**, removal of the '**β-strand insert**' (γ381–390) from its central domain. The '**β-strand insert**' (**black arrow**) is a part of the β-sheet structure located in the central domain, panel **A**. It is located between two antiparallel β-strands and is contiguous with the carboxy-terminal segment, residues **γ391-411-COOH**, in which reside its Gln398/399 and Lys406 cross-linking sites. The **curved arrow** in panel **B** shows how the 'β-strand insert' can be removed ('**pulled out'**) from the central domain to extend the carboxy-terminal segment, enabling it to undergo FXIII-catalyzed cross-linking with another carboxy-terminal γ-segment [Reproduced from Yakovlev S, Litvinovich S, Loukinov D, Medved L. Ann NY Acad Sci. 936:122-124, 2001]. I inserted another representation of pullout and transverse γ chain positioning in Leonid Medved's bio-sketch (Chapter 11).*

Siebenlist's Brainchild

In 2000, *Kevin Siebenlist* [22] and I reported on experiments that exploited the size differences between γA chains (/) and variant γ′ chains (( ) [23]. We mixed *radioactively* labeled γA–γ′ *fibrin* with *non-radioactive* γA-γA *fibrinogen* and then added FXIII to promote cross-linking of the fibrin-fibrinogen components (Figure 11). SDS gel-electrophoretic analyses of the disulfide-reduced mixtures yielded equal amounts of two discrete radioactive dimer bands corresponding to γA–γA and γA–γ′, in exactly the amounts predicted for fibrinogen/fibrin molecules undergoing cross-linking of *transversely* positioned γ chains.

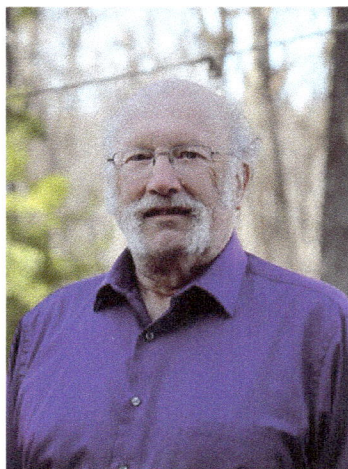

Had the mixture of radioactive γA–γ′ fibrin and non-radioactive γA-γA fibrinogen possessed *longitudinally* positioned carboxy-terminal γ chain segments, that arrangement would have produced monomeric radioactive monomeric γA and γ′ chains and non-radioactive γA-γA dimers. Such entities *did not* appear and therefore they do *not* exist!

Siebenlist's findings were as convincing and irrefutable as any of our previous reports, and they did *not* involve any electron microscopy. Despite this, Russ Doolittle carelessly or perhaps willfully, lumped our report with several others as *"opposing electron microscopic observations"* in

---

[22] Kevin Siebenlist has been my colleague and associate since he joined my group in 1984. His contributions were chronicled in the first volume of *Fibrinogen Memoirs* and several of them are restated in this volume. Kevin began post-graduate studies at the Medical College of Wisconsin in the MD-PhD program, but after a short time in a dual capacity he dropped the MD program and opted to complete the PhD program in Biochemistry. After obtaining that degree he joined my research group. Our collegial and collaborative relationship still exists and includes him being a loyal golf partner.

his paper on X-ray crystallographic studies of fibrinogen and fibrin [21]. He dismissed all of them without explanation.

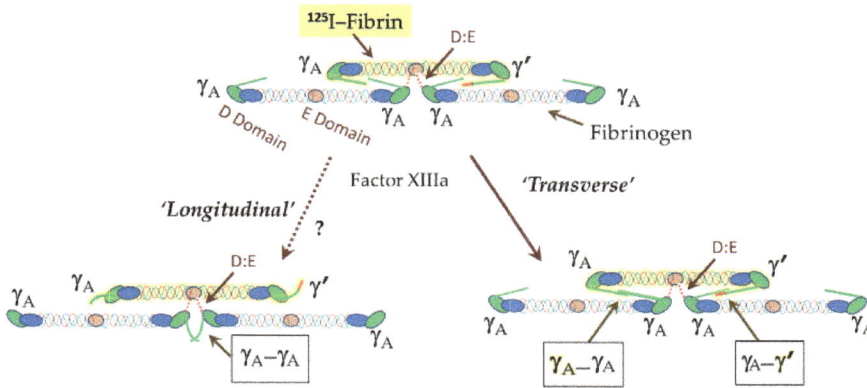

Figure 11. *The protocol for distinguishing 'longitudinal' (**left dotted arrow**) from 'transverse' γ-γ chain positioning (**right arrow**). The fibrin-fibrinogen mixtures were composed of radioactive γA–γ' fibrin and non-radioactive γA–γA fibrinogen. The radioactive γ dimer species we found are highlighted in* yellow *(**lower right**). **Non-radioactive** γA-γA dimers (**lower left**) would have been found if longitudinal cross-link positioning existed. **None** was found!*

Chapter 13
The Debate and a Failed Collaboration

In 2003, *Robert Ariens,* an Associate Editor of The Journal of Thrombosis and Hemostasis, invited me and John Weisel to engage in a written debate about the γ chain cross-linking issue. The articles appeared in 2004 [24,25] and were followed by rebuttal statements [26,27].

Among the diagrams included in my narrative was one that illustrated the consequences of maximally stretching a *transversely* cross-linked fibrin fibril. I have here updated that diagram (Figure 12) to better illustrate how this arrangement accounts for elastic recovery. The

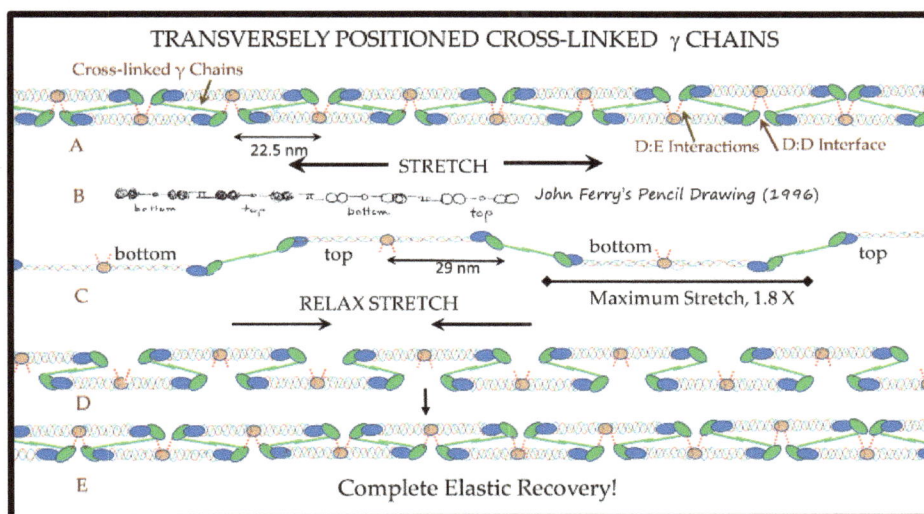

Figure 12. *This drawing illustrates what would happen to the structure of a transversely cross-linked fibrin fibril [A] when stretched to its limit (1.8 X and 29 nm periodicity, Ferry's estimate), [B,C] and how it would recover its original form after the strain had been released [D,E]. The pencil drawing by John Ferry showing 'top' and 'bottom' molecules [B] are identified in the stretched fibril drawing below it [C]. In a transverse configuration, cross-linked γ chains would behave like springs that return the stretched fibril to its original shape. Terminology is the same as in Fig. 1.*

'lattice-like' arrangement of transversely cross-linked γ chains allows them to function like 'springs' that return a stretched fibrin polymer to its original shape. There are other structures in the fibrin network, *trimolecular junctions,*[23] that likely contribute to the elastic properties of fibrin, but at this *juncture* (pun intended) we can only conjecture about their role in this process.

The *longitudinal* cross-link configuration championed by Weisel, Doolittle, and others, cannot fulfill the theoretical requirements that are needed for elasticity recovery of a fibrin polymer (Figure 13), since that particular configuration would lack the *inter*-fibril strand connections that are known to exist in cross-linked fibrin. If a *longitudinal* arrangement existed, when strain was imposed upon such a structure, the stretched fibril strands would slide past one another and the polymer would thereby undergo *inelastic 'viscous' deformation,* as illustrated below. Such deformation does *not* occur in cross-linked fibrin clots. In further support of that logic, it is needless to reiterate that there is a mountain of evidence supporting *transverse* cross-link positioning, and not even one study offering credible evidence for the *longitudinal* cross-link arrangement.

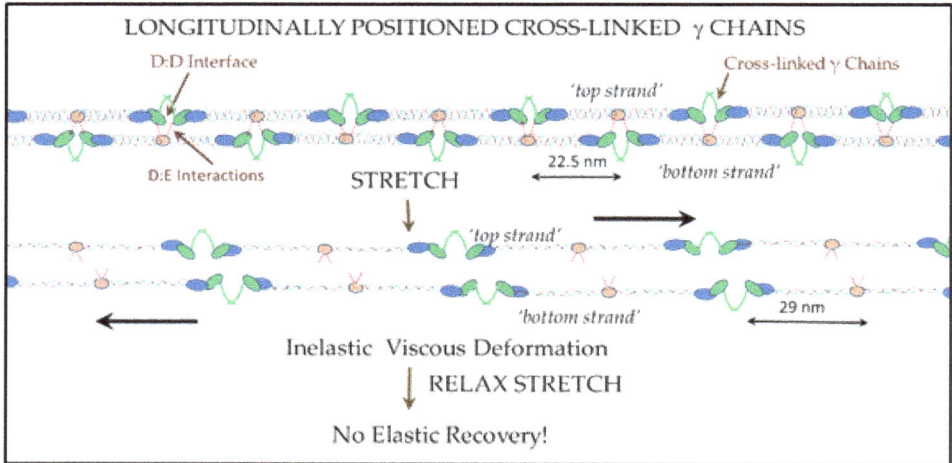

Figure 13. Drawing of a 'longitudinally' cross-linked fibrin fibril, illustrating what would occur when such a structure was subjected to strain. In this drawing, non-covalent D:E connections are disrupted as 'top' and 'bottom' fibril strands slide past one another. A bond arrangement like this could not support elastic recovery.

---

[23] There is a chapter in *Fibrinogen Memoirs* on the discovery and characterization of these branch points [1]. [Also see *Addendum 10.*]

The Rebuttals

In rebuttal arguments I further deconstructed Weisel's flawed protocols, rationales, and arguments. I emphasized the facts that he had ignored, denied, or misrepresented. I further defended what I believed my own airtight argument for a *transverse* arrangement.

In his own rebuttal, Weisel presented an alternative reality. He denied the validity of evidence showing that *longitudinal* cross-linking does not occur in assembled fibrin fibrils and couched his denial with elliptical statements about 'conformation'. When it came to the 'pull out' hypothesis, for which Yakovlev et al. had presented unassailable evidence, Weisel's response was simply: *"No evidence for the 'pull-out' hypothesis"*. With those statements he had abandoned facts and logic.

He also suggested that plasmic degradation products produced from *longitudinally* cross-linked fibrin were somehow qualitatively different from those that form from *transversely* cross-linked fibrin, a subject we had debated for years without resolution.

Evidence from STEM images and quantitative analyses of ligated D-fibrin-D complexes under selected solvent conditions [12], showed that non-covalent D:E bonds were critically important for determining the position of cross-linked γ chains in fibrin fibrils. *John Weisel* dismissed these results using an argument derived from his mistaken beliefs on the nature of cross-linked fibrin degradation products. He also mistook my conjecture about the connection between *transverse* cross-linking and fibrin elasticity, to be evidentiary, an interpretation that I did not anticipate.

In my narrative I also presented a soliloquy on the relationship between *transversely* cross-linked fibrin and the elastic properties of cross-linked fibrin, the role that *John Ferry* had played in fostering that idea, and the 'group-think' that had collectively ratified such a conjecture. I also reasoned that *longitudinally* cross-linked fibrin, owing to the unfavorable positioning of cross-linked γ chains within fibril strands, could not confer elasticity to fibrin, as reviewed at the beginning of this chapter (see Figures 12, 13). It was my strong belief then as now, that the relationship between fibrin structure and its elasticity was an unavoidable scenario.

As considered in the next chapter, I discovered two investigations that emerged during the decade that followed our debate that inadvertently and unwittingly had supported my conclusions [29, 30].[24]

One More Experiment?

A few weeks after the Debate articles had been published, *Paul Bishop* paid me a visit at the Blood Research Institute (BRI). Paul worked at Zymogenetics, a biopharmaceutical company that under his guidance, had produced and marketed recombinant Factor XIII. He was well versed on the cross-linking controversy, a subject we had previously discussed in detail. During our meeting, he excitedly told me about an experimental protocol that he had devised that could distinguish unambiguously between *transverse* and *longitudinal* arrangements. This was how he described it (illustrations are mine):

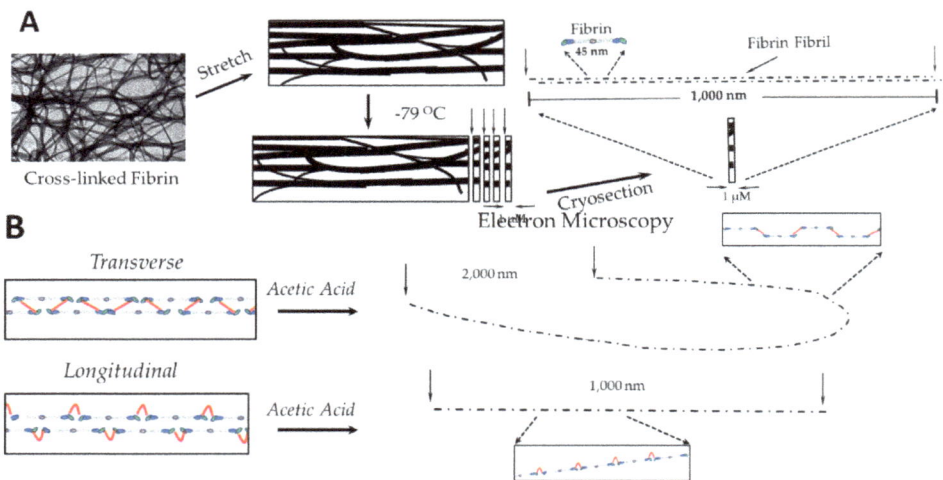

1) Prepare a cross-linked fibrin clot (Panel 'A', *left section)*; orient the fibers in a parallel plane by stretching (*middle sections)*; 2) Freeze the stretched specimen in dry ice (-79°C), then prepare sagittal sections of uniform width in the frozen state in a Cryostat. If the width of each slice was 1 μM

---

[24] *Litvinov* and *Weisel* were co-authors of reference '29'. They probably did not realize that evidence presented in that paper supported a direct relationship between *transverse* γ chain cross-linking and fibrin *elasticity*, an oversight that reinforces the regret that I expressed over investigations that have failed to consider their results in terms of a *transverse* cross-linking arrangement.

(1,000 nm), each double-stranded fibril section in the slice would contain ~44 fibrin molecules (each per 45 *nm*).[25] (Panel 'B', *right section*). **3**) Pool the frozen slices, suspend them in acetic acid solutions to *dissociate* non-covalent D:E interactions, then examine the single-stranded products by Electron Microscopy (Panel 'B', *right section).* Single strands derived from *transversely* cross-linked fibrils (*left section, upper*) will have a contour length twice that of strands derived from *longitudinally* cross-linked fibrils (*left section, lower*), in this case 2,000 nm versus 1,000 nm. The value to determine would be the ratio of 'strand length' ÷ 'section width'. A ratio of 2:1 would indicate that these strands originated from '*transversely*' cross-linked fibrils whereas a ratio of 1:1 would indicate a '*longitudinally*' cross-linked fibril origin.

I congratulated Paul for designing such a clever and potentially useful protocol, one that might well add to the existing body of evidence for *transverse* cross-linking. We then switched our discussion to other subjects and the meeting ended. I wrote down my recollections of Bishop's protocol and filed it in a desk drawer. I had no interest at that time of undertaking yet another experiment to prove what I had already proven to my own satisfaction.

A few months later *John Weisel* came to The Blood Research Institute (BRI) to deliver an invited Research Seminar on a subject not related to cross-linking. I was his host, of course. During the visit, as usual, we discussed the cross-linking issue at length. It was clear that John had not altered his position and, if anything, was even more hostile to my ideas than ever before. Then, I remembered *Paul Bishop's* protocol! It had features that lent themselves to a joint project, and '*collaboration*' was exactly what I had in mind. The experiment, if successful, could unambiguously distinguish between the two cross-linking schemes. It

---

[25] Calculation of the number of fibrin molecules in a 1 μM section of a double-stranded fibril: $1,000\ nm\ \div\ 45\ nm\ per\ fibrin\ molecule\ \text{X}\ 2\ strands\ per\ fibril = \mathbf{44}$ molecules. A covalently linked single strand derived from a *longitudinally* cross-linked fibril would contain 22 molecules ($1,000 \div 45\ \text{X}\ 1 = 22$), whereas the single strands derived from a *transversely* cross-linked fibril would contain 44 molecules! The ratio of strand length per μM (i.e., 2:1 versus 1:1) would unambiguously distinguish between a *transverse* and a *longitudinal* cross-linking arrangement.

seemed like a golden opportunity to bring Weisel into my camp at last. I had no idea whether my proposal would pose an unbearable threat to his immutable fixation on the *longitudinal* cross-link arrangement, but it was worth a try.

To make the experiment even more attractive, I modified Bishop's protocol to make it more foolproof than it already was. In addition to using 'off the shelf' 'intact' fibrinogen that Bishop's protocol called for, I proposed using *Des /α fibrinogen*,[4] as the fibrin substrate for cross-linking. Des /α fibrinogen (aka, Fraction I-9) contains truncated Aα chains that lack cross-linking sites, a feature would eliminate any potential confounding effects from concomitant cross-linking of α chains.

In addition, Weisel possessed a 'one-of-a-kind' apparatus for orienting network fibers in a parallel plane in a magnetic field. Not only would use of his apparatus eliminate any possible distortions that might occur under stretching conditions (Panel A), but more importantly it would deepen the co-dependency of our collaboration. For my part of the collaboration, I would undertake frozen sectioning of magnetically oriented fibrin specimens in a Cryostat and return the pooled slices to him for Electron Microscopic analysis in his laboratory. The latter part was important to me since I wanted him to make the critical observations and measurements. During that period, I helped him to establish buffer and cross-linking conditions by carrying out pilot analyses at the BNL STEM facility After considering my proposal, he happily agreed to the collaboration, and off we went!

The project advanced in the weeks and months that followed. I sent him intact fibrinogen, des /α fibrinogen, and Factor XIII. Together, we set the solvent and imaging conditions. Eventually he prepared magnetically oriented cross-linked fibrin specimens and shipped them to me for thin sectioning. As we had agreed, I cryo-sectioned the specimens in 1 μM slices, pooled and suspended the slices and shipped the material to him for further analysis.

I withheld a small amount of the cryo-sectioned product and had it imaged under non-dissociating buffer conditions by STEM at the Brookhaven facility. When I reviewed the STEM images, among fields of aggregated material, I identified double-stranded 'fibrils' ~1 µM in length. These observations suggested that we were on the right track.

I did not examine the specimen under dissociating solvent conditions that would have allowed imaging of single strands because I wanted Weisel to make those observations himself, but I did inform him of my preliminary findings.

I didn't hear much from him for a few weeks, and when I finally did, he informed me that despite extensive and time-consuming efforts, he had encountered significant difficulties in establishing cross-linking conditions for magnetically oriented specimens. He was also concerned with other potential 'artefacts' that might complicate the results. John did not report having tried to image the cross-linked cryo-sectioned specimens that I had sent to him earlier. He also informed me that he would have to pay more attention to his grant-related studies and other pressing matters. After that unsatisfying exchange, our communications became less frequent and less forthcoming. Eventually, my enthusiasm petered out, and that turned out to be an unceremonious end to what had once been a promising collaboration. After that, we did not discuss any aspect of our collaboration again and I was left to wonder about what the outcome of this project might have been.

Chapter 14
Becoming A Myth–2005 to 2020

Following publication of the Debate articles and the Rebuttals there was a dearth of reports dealing with the cross-linking controversy. I contributed to those doldrums myself. Shortly after the collaborative project between John Weisel and me ended, my interests turned in other directions. I still believed that additional experiments on cross-linking arrangements were unnecessary for there to be an airtight argument for a *transverse* arrangement.

I was unable to attend The Fibrinogen Workshop that took place in the UK in 2006. A few weeks after the conference had ended, I learned from several attendees, later confirmed by *John Weisel*, that an informal *ad hoc* session on cross-linking arrangements had taken place. It was a *False Flag* operation conducted by *Mattia Rocco* who, lacking license or insight, had solicited a 'vote' from the audience on which cross-linking arrangement was correct. As transmitted in a letter to me written by Weisel, Rocco asked him to let me know that "*transverse* cross-linking had lost!".

I was angrily surprised and discouraged to learn about that event, since it had been orchestrated in my absence by someone with a severely limited understanding of the issues involved, someone who had never made any substantive scientific contributions of his own on that subject. I expressed my concerns to Mattia who apologized to me and then tried to pass it off as a joke. He did not recognize how hurtful it had been coming from someone who was so ill informed. Additional discussions between us did not assuage me or change my opinion about his behavior.

Despite that disappointment, I continued to follow literature related to the cross-linking controversy until 2010, when I read the report

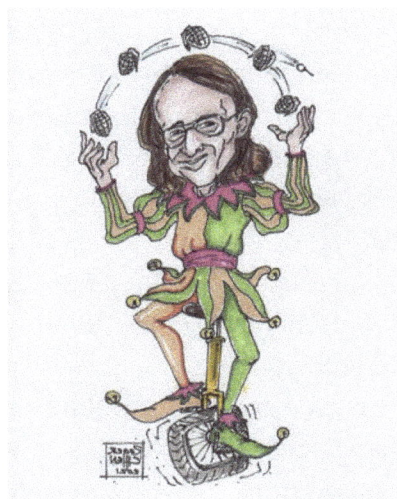

73

from *Martin Guthold's* group concerning the mechanical properties of stretched and cross-linked single fibrin fibers [3]. Their report had finessed the controversy altogether by making the unqualified assumption that a *longitudinal* bond arrangement existed in cross-linked fibrin. There was no qualifying explanation or relevant literature citation.

I was discouraged by their failure and when added to other recent and more remote events, I decided to divert my attention from that subject entirely, in effect a self-applied leave-of-absence that lasted for a decade.

My absence lasted until just after I had signed off on publication of the first volume of *Fibrinogen Memoirs* in August 2020. During that same month, an Email message from the publishing company, *Elsevier*, reached my Inbox. The email promoted a 2017 issue of *Matrix Biology* that was devoted to 'Fibrin and Fibrinogen'. Among the subjects covered in the issue was an article by *Litvinov and Weisel* [5] that reviewed recent advances in measuring and modeling the mechanical properties of fibrin polymers. After a thorough reading, it was clear to me that the *transverse* cross-linking arrangement was on the 'endangered species' list, in imminent danger of becoming a Myth. With that realization I ended my self-imposed boycott.

Among other items, their review referenced a more recent study from *Guthold's* laboratory [28] which had doubled down on their earlier presumption of *longitudinal* cross-link location and as a consequence, had also proposed that longitudinally connected D-D domains were *"Rigid D:D interactions"*. That was a frivolous speculation leading to the unlikely conclusion that *"the αC region is largely responsible for the elasticity, strain hardening, and large strains in the mechanical behavior of fibrin fibers."*

Other studies cited by Litvinov and Weisel had focused on biomechanical properties of fibrin. Each had assumed *longitudinal* cross-link positioning as a given feature of the polymer. That same assumption was true as well for publications that appeared after the Litvinov article had been published, even when their findings contradicted that assumption. These are considered in the next section.

Unwitting Support for Transverse Cross-linking

Zhmurov et al. [29] carried out *'forced unfolding'* experiments using AFM (Atomic Force Microscopy) on cross-linked *fibrinogen* oligomers formed from *des /α-fibrinogen*, a subfraction lacking α chain cross-linking sites.[26] The unfolding pattern of the oligomers formed from *des /α-fibrinogen* was indistinguishable from those formed from *intact* fibrinogen preparations containing a full measure of αC cross-linking sites. Based on their findings, Zhmurov et al. concluded: *"molecular elongation is determined by combined sequential unfolding transitions in the C-terminal γ chain nodules and limited reversible extension-contraction of the α-helical coiled-coil connectors"*. Although not explicitly stated, their conclusion confirmed ours on formation of *cross-linked fibrinogen fibrils* [13], a study that had provided unassailable evidence for a *transverse* arrangement of cross-linked γ chains. Their measurements also confirmed that *transversely* positioned cross- linked γ chains account for fibrin's *elasticity*.[27]

Duval et al. [30], in studies of cross-linking and fibrin *elasticity*, compared a recombinant fibrinogen (γQ_{398-9}, K_{406} –'3X') that was not capable of undergoing γ chain cross-linking, with 'wild type' fibrinogen, '**WT**. In the absence of FXIII, WT fibrin developed a higher *'storage modulus'* than 3X, a finding that *"reflects the elastic energy stored during deformation"* (i.e., *elasticity*). When FXIII was included in the mixtures, cross-linked WT fibrin was less susceptible to viscous deformation compared to 3X. These results indicated that cross-linking of γ *chains* played a *major* role in conferring fibrin *elasticity*. The experimental protocols upon which Duval et al. based their conclusions were 'complimentary' to those used by *Zhmurov*, in that both investigated the

---

[26] I provided *des /α-fibrinogen* to these investigators for experiments showing that this *fibrinogen* subfraction formed *oligomers,* a result that confirmed our prior observations on *cross-linked fibrinogen fibrils [13]* (also see Chapter 10). Their results confirmed ours and demonstrated that *transverse* positioning of cross-linked γ chains accounts for formation of fibrinogen oligomers!

[27] *Litvinov* and *Weisel* were co-authors of the *Zhmurov* paper. They will surely be aghast when they realize that they co-signed a report providing confirmatory evidence for *transverse* positioning of cross-linked γ chains!

same fibrinogen functionalities (or the absence thereof). In both instances they arrived at the same conclusions.[28]

In a later study on the same subject (2018), Zhmurov et al. examined cross-linked fibrin with 'high resolution' AFM [31]. Although they were unable to resolve the carboxy-terminal regions of γ chains with that technique, [29] they arbitrarily chose to position those segments *'longitudinally'* between the abutting D Domains that formed each strand of a fibril. That assignment was consistent with the 'party line' espoused by their co-author, *John Weisel*. By choosing this cross-linking construct, they disregarded their earlier results (discussed above) on 'forced unfolding' of fibrinogen oligomers [29], that had led to the alternative conclusion.

Befuddling Reports

Koenderink's group contributed several reports on the biomechanical properties of fibrin. Among these, Kumiawan et al. [32] laudably noted that cross-linking was responsible for suppressing viscous deformation. Further analysis of this process then fell short because they only considered α-polymers in modeling their findings. The only mention of γ chain cross-linking was "within and between", a confusing phrase.

In another offering, Pierchocka et al. [33] determined the elastic properties of recombinant fibrin and found that γ chain cross-linking contributed to *clot elasticity* by changing the 'force-extension' behavior of the 'protofibrils', whereas α-chain cross-linking stiffens the fibers because of 'tighter coupling' between constituent fibrils. That conclusion is

---

[28] *Robert Ariens* was a co-author of the *Duval* paper [30] and also had been the Editor for the 2004 'Debates'. In those times past he told me that he favored the *longitudinal* cross-linking arrangement because *"Nature is Parsimonious"*. [2]. I queried him again more recently about his preference given the exculpatory findings in the *Duval* study. He wrote back that his preference for a *longitudinal* arrangement had not changed.

[29] Image resolution with AFM was lower than that with STEM. In our prior investigation using STEM, we located *transversely* oriented crossed-linked γ chain regions in assembled fibrinogen fibrils as filaments bridging between fibril strands [13]. In another set of experiments, we located electron dense Au_{11} tagged carboxy-termini of γ chains in fibrinogen and in fibrin fibrils. We found most of the Au_{11} particles between the D and E Domains of molecules [19], as related in Chapter 12.

problematic since they positioned cross-linked γ chains between the D Domains of fibrin molecules in each strand, in the *'longitudinal'* arrangement. If instead, had they considered the *'lattice-like'* arrangement of *transversely* positioned cross-linked γ chains, they might have recognized that this was the *only* arrangement that could support fibrin elasticity.

Vos et al. [34] used *in situ* small angle X-Ray scattering to investigate fibrin elastometric behavior at a molecular level. They "channeled" the γ-γ crosslinks as positioned *"along the 'longitudinal' direction of the monomer"*, as posited by *Guthold's* group [28], *"which may channel stress through the D and E nodules and the coiled coils"*. They diagrammed their speculations and conclusions in the drawing shown in Figure 14. In their diagram, 'protofibrils' consisted of "2 or 3 fibrin units

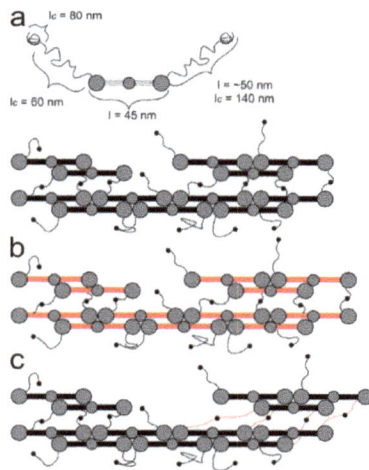

Figure 14. *From Vos et al. [34]."**a**) A fibrin monomer **(above)** with extended αC-regions"*. *"(below) Sections of two connected protofibrils at rest"*. *"The packing defect in the top row arises due to the finite length of the protofibrils"*. *"(**b,c**) Schematic representation of two elongation mechanisms for fibrin fibers"*, *"**b**, through forced unfolding of the monomer"*, *"**c**, through entropic stretching of the natively unfolded αC-connectors"*.

of finite length" and they proposed that elongation resulting from strain was a function of 'coiled coil' elongation (Figure 13, '**b**', red areas). They believed that their measurements "strongly support earlier proposals that reversible stretching of the αC regions plays an important role in fiber elongation". It was difficult to relate these statements to their representations of assembled fibrils. Because *John Weisel* co-signed this publication, I defer to him on dealing with that problem.

Chapter 15

Perspectives and Conclusions

In the preceding chapter, I reviewed reports appearing between 2010 and 2020 that were concerned with fibrin biomechanical properties, and that had collectively contributed to the transition of the cross-linking controversy to a myth. I divided the articles into two cross-linking 'baskets', *Transverse* and *Longitudinal*, depending on the evidence presented. Two reports fell into the *Transverse* basket [29, 30]. Both of these studies provided evidence that *transversely* cross-linked γ chains conferred elasticity to fibrin, although they did reach the same conclusion. In addition, the *Zhmurov* study [29] also contained confirmatory evidence for a *transverse* cross-linked γ chain arrangement. Neither report, however, interpreted their findings in terms of a *'longitudinal'* or *'transverse'* cross-linking construct, but since fibrin elasticity depends on the formation of cross-linked γ chains, their findings, *pari passu*, show that *transverse* cross-link positioning accounts for fibrin's *elastic* behavior.

The other studies cited in that chapter fell into the *'Longitudinal'* basket. Each had implied or tacitly assumed that there was a *longitudinal* cross-linking arrangement in fibrin. None of them provided any tangible evidence, literature citation, or discussion to support that assumption. With the exception of the report by Zhmurov et al. [22], none of them acknowledged that a controversy about fibrin cross-linking had even existed. When coupled with other studies that appeared during the past decade, I aver that *transverse* cross-linking and the 'Cross-linking Controversy', have become a *Myth*.

The desire to write about some of my life's experiences and review my scientific accomplishments and failures, motivated me to write the first volume of *Fibrinogen Memoirs*. Its sequel came about for a different reason, namely, realization that the concept of a *transverse* cross-linking arrangement had fallen into undeserved disrepute and disuse in favor of the other cross-linking scheme, *longitudinal*, for which I could not find any credible supporting evidence. I was determined to address that oversight and the only way to do this was to write this sequel, *Fibrinogen Memoirs– The Rise and Fall of the Fibrin Cross-linking Controversy*.

I also tried to understand and attempted to explain '*how*' this situation came about. One possible explanation I can offer is that by overlooking the existence of the *transverse* cross-linking scheme, it became easier to take a simpler, more familiar path of least resistance, and thereby be enabled to ignore an uncomfortable and inconvenient truth.

Much of the personal responsibility for the demise of the *transverse* cross-linking arrangement and the controversy itself, should rest with my erstwhile colleague, *John Weisel*. During the entire period that the controversy existed, he never once seemed able to grasp the flaws in his own experimental designs and he never understood why the conclusions drawn by *Russ Doolittle* were unsupportable. In that connection, Doolittle, because of well-deserved notoriety, and unflinching persuasiveness, played an equally important role.

Between 2010 and 2020 Weisel and his coworkers and collaborators published several reports, all of which proffered only the *longitudinal* cross-linking arrangement. *Weisel's* name on those publications signaled tacit or overt submission by all investigators, even when the results of their experiments indicated otherwise. I believe that John seems to have long since settled this issue in his own mind, and by co-signing studies which genuflected to his belief, he was enabled to reinforce earlier conclusions. That's the *how*!

Unpeeling the '*why*' of this situation is more difficult. The history of science is filled with 'Zombie' opposition to new ideas and discoveries. It is often a matter of accepting the easiest explanation and choosing the most traveled road. *Parsimony* was the word used by my colleague *Robert Ariens* to explain why he preferred a *longitudinal* arrangement. Perhaps the '*why*' is exemplified by what the Belgian playwright, poet, and Nobel Laureate in Literature (1911), *Maurice Maeterlinck* (1862-1949} wrote: "*At every crossroad on the path that leads to the future, tradition has placed against each of us ten thousand men to guard the past.*"

October 2021

Literature Citations

1. FIBRINOGEN MEMOIRS–JOURNEYS OF A CLOT DOCTOR. Mosesson, MW. *IPBooks, NY, Pub.* 1-247, 2020.

2. FIBRIN, THE PERFECT BIOELASTOMER. Mosesson, MW. In *Fibrinogen Memoirs–Journeys of A Clot Doctor.* Mosesson, MW. *IPBooks, NY, Pub.* 2020, p. 77-104.

3. THE MECHANICAL PROPERTIES OF SINGLE FIBRIN FIBERS. Liu W, Carlisle CR, Sparks EA, Guthold M. *J Thromb Haemostas* 8:1030-6, 2010

4. SHORT BY ONE MECHANISM. [Letter to the Editor]. Mosesson MW. *J Thromb Haemostas* 8:2089, 2010.

5. FIBRIN MECHANICAL PROPERTIES AND THEIR STRUCTURAL ORIGINS. Litvinov RI, Weisel JW. *Matrix Biol* 60-61:110-123, 2017.

6. STRUCTURAL ASPECTS OF THE FIBRINOGEN TO FIBRIN CONVERSION. Doolittle RF. *Adv Protein Chem* 27:1-109, 1973.

7. CROSSLINKED FIBRINOGEN DIMERS DEMONSTRATE A FEATURE OF THE MOLECULAR PACKING IN FIBRIN FIBERS. Fowler WE, Erickson HP, Hantgan RR, McDonagh J, Hermans J. *Science* 211:287-9, 1981.

8. CROSSLINKING OF FIBRINOGEN TO IMMOBILIZED DES AA FIBRIN. Selmayr E, Thiel W, Müller-Berghaus G. *Thromb Res* 39:459-65, 1985.

9. CHROMATOGRAPHY AND ELECTRON MICROSCOPY OF CROSS-LINKED FIBRIN POLYMERS--A NEW MODEL DESCRIBING THE CROSS-LINKING AT THE DD-TRANS CONTACT OF THE FIBRIN MOLECULES. Selmayr E, Deffner M, Bachmann L, Müller-Berghaus G. *Biopolymers* 27:1733-48, 1988.

10. IDENTIFICATION OF COVALENTLY LINKED TRIMEERIC AND TETRAMERIC D DOMAINS IN CROSSLINKED FIBRIN. Mosesson MW, Siebenlist KR, Amrani DL, DiOrio JP. *Proc Natl Acad Sci (USA)* 86:1113-7, 1989.

11. DETERMINATION OF THE TOPOLOGY OF FACTOR XIIIA-INDUCED FIBRIN γ-CHAIN CROSS-LINKS BY ELECTRON MICROSCOPY OF LIGATED FRAGMENTS. Weisel JW, Francis CW, Nagaswani C, Marder VJ. *J Biol Chem* 268:26618-24, 1993.

12. ORIENTATION OF THE CARBOXY-TERMINAL REGIONS OF FIBRIN γ CHAIN DIMERS DETERMIINED FROM THE CROSSLINKED

PRODUCTS FORMED IN MIXTURES OF FIBRIN, FRAGMENT D, AND FACTOR XIIIa. Siebenlist KR, Meh DA, Wall JS, Hainfeld JF, Mosesson MW. *Thromb Haemostas* 74:1113-9, 1995.

13. THE COVALENT STRUCTURE OF FACTOR XIIIa CROSSLINKED FIBRINOGEN FIBRILS. Mosesson MW, Siebenlist KR, Hainfeld JF, Wall JS. *J Struct Biol* 115:G88-101, 1995.

14. PROTRANSGLUTAMINASE (FACTOR XIII) MEDIATED CROSSLINKING OF FIBRINOGEN AND FIBRIN. Siebenlist KR, Meh DA, Mosesson MW. *Thromb Haemostas* 86:1221-8, 2001.

15. CRYSTAL STRUCTURES OF FRAGMENT D FROM HUMAN FIBRINOGEN AND ITS CROSSLINKED COUNTERPART FROM FIBRIN. Spraggon G, Everse SJ, Doolittle RF. *Nature* 389:455-62, 1997.

16. THE COMPLEMENTARY AGGREGATION SITES OF FIBRIN INVESTIGATED THROUGH EXAMINATION OF POLYMERS OF FIBRINOGEN WITH FRAGMENT E. Veklich YI, Ang EK, Lorand L, Weisel JW. *Proc Natl Acad Sci USA* 95:1438-42, 1998.

17. A DOUBLE-HEADED GLY-PRO-ARG-PRO LIGAND MIMICS THE FUNCTIONS OF THE E DOMAIN OF FIBRIN FOR PROMOTING THE END-TO-END CROSSLINKING OF γ CHAINS BY FACTOR XIIIa. Lorand, L, Parameswaran KN, Prasanna Murthy SN. *Proc Natl Acad Sci USA* 95:537-541, 1998.

18. FIBRINOGEN ASSEMBLY AND CROSSLINKING ON A FIBRIN FRAGMENT E TEMPLATE. Mosesson MW, Siebenlist KR, Hernandez I, Wall JS, Hainfeld JF. *Thromb Haemostas* 87:651-658, 2002.

19. THE LOCATION OF THE CARBOXY-TERMINAL REGION OF GAMMA CHAINS IN FIBRINOGEN AND FIBRIN D DOMAINS. Mosesson, MW, Siebenlist KR, Meh DA, Wall JS, Hainfeld, JF. *Proc Natl Acad Sci USA* 95:10511-6, 1998.

20. ROLE OF THE BETA-STRAND INSERT IN THE CENTRAL DOMAIN OF THE FIBRINOGEN GAMMA-MODULE. Yakovlev S, Litvinovich S, Loukinov D, Medved L. *Biochemistry* 39:15721-9, 2000.

21. X-RAY CRYSTALLOGRAPHIC STUDIES ON FIBRINOGEN AND FIBRIN. Doolittle RF. *J Thromb Haemost* 1:1559-65, 2003.

22. STRUCTURAL BASIS OF INTERFACIAL FLEXIBILITY IN FIBRIN OLIGOMERS. Zhmurov A, Protopopova AD, Litvinov RI, Zhukov P, Mukhitov AR, Weisel JW, Barsegov V. *Structure* 24:1907-17, 2016

23. POSITION OF γ CHAIN CARBOXY-TERMINAL REGIONS IN FIBRINOGEN-FIBRIN CROSSLINKING MIXTURES. Siebenlist KR, Meh DA, Mosesson MW. *Biochemistry* 39:14171-5, 2000.

24. THE FIBRIN CROSS-LINKING DEBATE: CROSS-LINKED GAMMA-

CHAINS IN FIBRIN FIBRILS BRIDGE 'TRANSVERSELY' BETWEEN STRANDS: YES. Mosesson MW. *J Thromb Haemost* 2:388-93, 2004.

25. THE FIBRIN CROSS-LINKING DEBATE: CROSS-LINKED GAMMA-CHAINS IN FIBRIN FIBRILS BRIDGE 'TRANSVERSELY' BETWEEN STRANDS: NO. Weisel JW. *Thromb Haemost* 2:394-9, 2004.

26. CROSS-LINKED GAMMA-CHAINS IN A FIBRIN FIBRIL ARE SITUATED TRANSVERSELY BETWEEN ITS STRANDS. Weisel JW. *J Thromb Haemost* 2:1467-9, 2004.

27. CROSS-LINKED GAMMA-CHAINS IN A FIBRIN FIBRIL ARE SITUATED TRANSVERSELY BETWEEN ITS STRANDS. Mosesson MW. *J Thromb Haemost* 2:1469-71, 2004.

28. A MODULAR FIBRINOGEN MODEL THAT CAPTURES THE STRESS-STRAIN BEHAVIOR OF FIBEIN FIBERS. Averett RD, Menn B, Lee EH, Helm CC, Barker T, Guthold M. *Biophys J* 103:1537-44, 2012.

29. MECHANISM OF FIBRIN(OGEN) FORCED UNFOLDING. Zhmurov A, Brown AEX, Litvinov RI, Weisel JW. *Structure* 19:1615-24, 2011.

30. ROLES OF FIBRIN α- AND γ-CHAIN SPECIFIC CROSS-LINKING BY FXIIIa IN FIBRIN STRUCTURE AND FUNCTION. Duval C, Connell SDA, Ridger VC, Philipou H, Ariëns RAS. *Thromb Haemostas* 111:842-50, 2014.

31. ATOMIC STRUCTURAL MODELS OF FIBRIN OLIGOMERS. Zhmurov A, Protopopova AD, Litvinov RI, Zhukov P, Weisel JW. *Structure* 26:857-68, 2018.

32. FIBRIN NETWORKS SUPPORT RECURRING MECHANICAL LOADS BY ADAPTING THEIR STRUCTURE ACROSS MULTIPLE SCALES. Kumiawan NA, Vos BA, Biebricher A, Wuite GJL, Peterman EJG, Koenderink GH. *Biophys J* 111:1026-34, 2016

33. RECOMBINANT FIBRINOGEN REVEALS THE DIFFERENTIAL ROLES OF α- AND γ- CHAIN CROSS-LINKING AND MOLECULAR HETEROGENEITY IN FIBRIN CLOT STAIN-STIFFENING. Pierchocka IK, Kurniawan NA, Koopman J, Koenderink GH. *J Thromb Haemostas* 159:38-49, 2017.

34. REVEALING THE MOLECULAR ORIGINS OF FIBRIN'S ELASTOMETRIC PROPERTIES BY *IN SITU* X-RAY SCATTERING. Vos BE, Martinez-Torres C, Burla F, Weisel JW, Koenderink GH. *Acta Biomaterialia* 104:39-2, 2020.

Documents and Notes

Addendum 1 (Chapter 6)

MWM Letter to John Weisel–August, 1993

UNIVERSITY OF WISCONSIN MEDICAL SCHOOL   *Milwaukee Clinical Campus*
Department of Medicine

August 12, 1993

John Weisel, Ph.D.
University of Pennsylvania
Department of Cell and
  Developmental Biology
The School of Medicine
Philadelphia, PA 19104-6058

Dear John:

I appreciate your thoughtfulness in sending me a draft of your paper on fibrin γ chain crosslinking. Thanks for all the reprints. I had copies of most of them, but not originals. I would like to take this opportunity to make some semi-random comments on your findings and conclusions, and I'd like to do this in a way that will result in us establishing a useful dialogue on the subject of fibrinogen in general and γ chain crosslinking in particular.

1. The logic of your statement on page 4 (Fig. 1C and D) that transversely crosslinked fibrils would be less efficiently dissolved than longitudinally crosslinked fibrils is difficult to understand, and the diagram does not clarify the situation. What is the basis for the assumption that different bonds would have to be broken for 'transverse' versus 'longitudinal'? Since the products of digestion produced by plasmin are the same for either situation, and since there is no evidence that the rate of fibrinolysis is changed by γ dimer formation, per se, plasmin cleavage of either type of crosslinked structure would yield exactly the same D-dimer and E products.

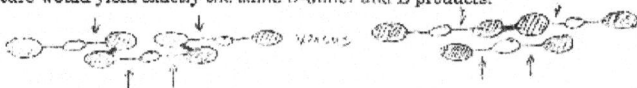

The evidence that Kevin presented in July at the ISTH meetings on fibrinolysis of crosslinked fibrin showed that resistance to fibrinolysis does not occur when only γ dimers have formed - therefore the rate (or efficiency as you put it) of dissolution is not changed by crosslinking at this level, whether longitudinal or transverse. As you may realize, the rate of fibrinolysis is substantially reduced as higher order γ chain crosslinks are formed (i.e., trimers, tetramers).

Affiliated with Sinai Samaritan Medical Center
945 North Twelfth St. P.O. Box 342
Milwaukee, Wisconsin 53201-0342

2. It appears to me that your experiments do not critically test whether longitudinal or transverse crosslinking occurs in fibrin. As I have tried to point out to anyone who will listen, crosslinked fibrinogen does not represent a satisfactory model for fibrin crosslinking since it may not necessarily assume the same configuration as an assembled crosslinked fibrin molecule. Is it not possible (or even likely) that the D-E interaction in fibrin plays a role in the configuration of the fibrin molecule D domain? Let us assume that the γ chain C-terminus can extend from the end of fibrinogen molecules.

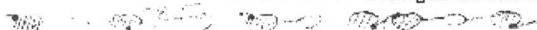

Thus, when they become crosslinked they align in an end-to-end fashion because there are no constraints to the positioning of the crosslinked D domain. But in an assembled fibrin matrix, this type of arrangement may occur -

a positioning brought about by the non-covalent D-E interaction. I'm not saying that I have direct evidence that this occurs, but I know of no reason why it cannot. [And there are the Selmayr experiments which suggest that it does.] The main point is this: when you disrupt non-covalent D-E interactions with denaturing solvents, the products are no longer constrained and are free to assume an elongated conformation such as occurs with crosslinked fibrinogen or fragment DY from crosslinked fibrin. Their appearance in the EM really does not test the question.

The argument about longitudinal versus transverse may be more semantic than real as it concerns fibril assembly. Kevin keeps pointing out to me that in a twisting fibril "end-to-end" may be effectively the same as "transverse" [see, for example, the highlighted molecules in attached Fig. 5 from Medved's paper in JMB]. In any case, if γ chain crosslinks can not bridge across fibrils and between fibrils how can γ trimers or γ tetramers ever form?

3. Fig. 2 - I don't understand why the "unfolded" fibrin fragments are drawn differently from the "longitudinal" ones. Why would the intermolecular D-D distance be any different in one form than in the other? [We have never observed D dimers, D trimers, or D tetramers in which the D domains were not close to one another, and neither, I suspect, have you.] Why would the "native" transverse be more likely to form "internal" D-E arrangements as opposed to "intermolecular" D-E arrangements? In any case, by disrupting non-covalent D-E interactions you lose the potential opportunity to distinguish that difference.

4. Fig. 4 - I assume that non-covalent D-E interactions tend to be dissociated in 30% glycerol and the volatile solvent you used. [In my experience, 30% glycerol dissociates non-crosslinked fibrin and therefore would probably disrupt D-E bonds.] Why then do double-stranded fibrils (bottom figure) occur if crosslinking is longitudinal and thus restricted to one or the other

strand in a two-stranded fibril?   What is the appearance of non-crosslinked fibrin or non crosslinked fibrin digests deposited under these conditions?

5. The Selmayr experiments (refs. 13-15) are difficult to explain away as some type of artifact (p.8). When we discovered the existence of γ trimers and γ tetramers, in order to account for these structures we hypothesized that γ chain crosslinking occurs across and between fibrils, at least some of the time. Putting that together with the Selmayr results led to our suggestions. We're hoping to provide an additional proof for that hypothesis, and expect to complete such an experiment (not an EM experiment) within the next few months. If it turns out that longitudinal crosslinking is the way that γ chains actually crosslink to one another, we'll then have to figure out how γ trimers and γ tetramers can form in a longitudinal crosslinking system.

6. p.10, line 3 ("With longitudinal...") I don't understand your statement regarding the expected appearance of transversely versus longitudinally crosslinked dimeric D structures [Are you assuming that "transverse" crosslinking creates a gap between D domains?]. I would not expect any differences in appearance irrespective of the crosslinking arrangement. The "lack of a gap" may demonstrate that the crosslinks are "longitudinal" in these structures but does not relate to the possible residual structures derived from transversely crosslinked fibrin.

I hope these comments give you a clear idea of the basis for my discontent with your conclusions. To whit, your results are consistent with the idea that γ chain crosslinking is longitudinal, and the images you've provided are excellent, but the results fall short, in my view, of proving such a structure. Furthermore, your proposal does not attempt to take into account the mechanism by which γ chain oligomers form, as they surely do.

I look forward to a continuing dialogue with you.

With best wishes.

Most sincerely,

Michael W. Mosesson, M.D.

MWM/ms

87

Fibrinogen Memoirs 2

Addendum 2 (Chapter 6)

John Weisel's Response -August, 1993

UNIVERSITY of PENNSYLVANIA

Department of
Cell and Developmental Biology
The School of Medicine
Philadelphia, PA 19104-6058
Tel: 215 898 8040
Fax 215 898-9871

August 23, 1993

Dr. Mike Mosesson
Department of Medicine
University of Wisconsin Medical School
Sinai Samaritan Medical Center
945 North Twelfth St. P.O. Box 342
Milwaukee 53201-0342

Dear Mike,

Thank you for your letter. I agree that it could be useful to establish a dialog on γ chain cross-linking and other aspects of fibrinogen. I will try to respond to all of the points that you raised.

1. I have included another copy of Fig. 1 with some markings to illustrate this point. Since DD/E complexes are normally produced by plasmin cleavage under physiological conditions, I have used orange lines mark off these DD/E complexes for the two cases. They cannot be the same because of the locations of the cross-links. As a result, the bonds at complementary binding sites (marked by red) must be broken for dissolution to occur with transverse cross-links. In other words, with longitudinal cross links plasmin cleavage easily results in formation of DD/E complex, while with transverse links that seems unlikely.

2. I agree with you completely that the earlier experiments with fibrinogen do not answer the critical question. That is why we did these experiments.

Your second point here that disruption of the non-covalent D-E contacts could allow the products to assume an elongated conformation is also a very good one. Since you had made this point at the ISTH meeting, I included this possibility in Fig. 2. As I have illustrated in Fig. 1 (similar to Selmayr, et al.'s diagram), the transverse model requires that there be a portion of the γ chain folded back toward the central part of the molecule. This part of the γ chain would be approximately 112 Å (1/4 of molecular length) long, but it could be considerably shorter (maybe as short as 65 Å). Thus, as you suggested, if this part of the molecule was not rigid, there could be an unfolding of the native conformation such that the fragments could appear to be elongated. In this case, there would probably be a wide variety structures of different appearances, but the most elongated ones would have the D regions separated by the length of two of these γ chain extensions. The important point is that experimentally we did not observe any examples with gaps between D regions. If there were transverse cross-links, it might be possible to find some examples like this, but it seems impossible for all fragments to undergo a transition from half-staggered to end-to-end. I do not see any way to account for these observations except the presence of longitudinal cross-links.

The example that you cite from our paper on protofibril structure appears to show some overlap of molecular ends. Although I hesitate to generalize from one example, this observation would be consistent with crystallographic results indicating some overlap (JMB **222** 89 (1991)). However, I would still call the interaction end-to-end or longitudinal. There are similar examples in other fields: e.g., tropomyosin interactions are called end-to-end, but they also exhibit a considerable molecular overlap.

As for your question of how to account for the presence of γ trimers and tetramers, as I suggested in my last letter, the simplest explanation would be that they occur between molecules of adjacent protofibrils as shown below:

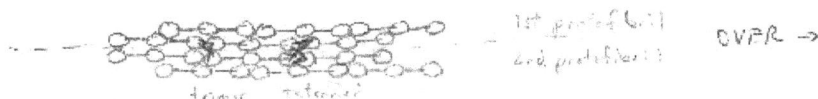

3. This question is discussed above. The main point is that the transverse model requires a γ chain extended toward the center of the molecule. Although there could be conformational changes in the presence of dilute acetic acid, I don't see any way to go from half-staggered to the appearance of end-to-end interactions with no gaps.

4. With our buffer conditions for these experiments, there is no (or negligible) disruption of non-covalent D-E interactions. In fact, we have followed polymerization of fibrin monomer to form oligomers under these conditions. It was necessary to use dilute acetic acid to dissociate the complexes into fragments. Therefore, Fig. 4 shows complexes, which are two-stranded structures.

5. I thought that the Selmayr experiments appeared convincing at first, but as described in our paper, when you examine them more closely there are some serious problems, especially the use of urea for electron microscope experiments. I also thought that your hypothesis about γ trimers and tetramers was a reasonable one, but now I think that they must occur across rather than within protofibrils.

6. The expected difference in appearance of the smaller fragments such as D dimer is related to the extended γ chain, as described above.

I hope that my reply answers your questions and clears up your discontent with our conclusions. You are correct that we have not accounted for the mechanism of formation of γ chain oligomers in the paper, but this paper does not deal with this question. I have given you my opinions, but for now, I would prefer to leave it to you to explain the mechanism of γ oligomers. My explanation here may be too simple-minded; you could probably do it better. I think that your experimental evidence is solid and do not see any major contradiction with longitudinal cross-linking (even though perhaps transverse cross-linking would have fit better). In any event, we can continue this dialog. Best wishes.

Sincerely yours,

John

John Weisel, Ph.D.

I just received reprints of our JMB paper & have included a few reprints

89

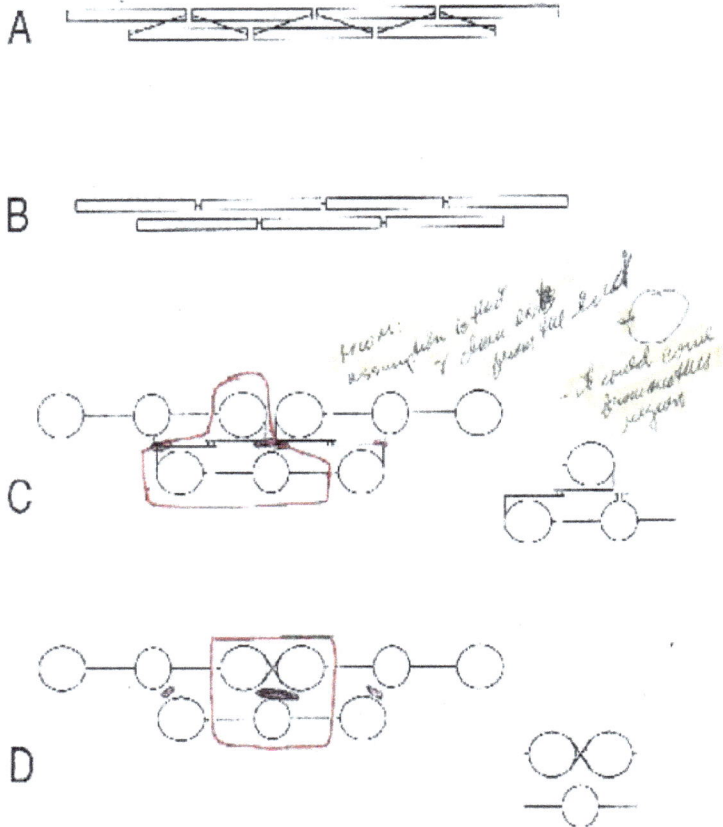

Figure 1 Weisel

Documents and Notes

Addendum 3 (Chapter 7)

Doolittle's mimeographed letter to his colleagues

November 1, 1969

PLEASE NOTE

We are writing to the hundreds of you who requested reprints or who received preprints of our recent article in PNAS (**reprint enclosed**) in order to draw your attention to two very recent articles by Dr. L. Lorand and his colleagues at Northwestern University. The developments leading to these latter publications warrant some elaboration.

Last April, having submitted our manuscript on the identification of the polypeptide chains involved in fibrin crosslinking to PNAS under the sponsorship of Professor Bruno Zimm (received April 7, 1969), we mailed preprints to about a dozen persons who we thought might find immediate benefit from our findings. The choice of these persons was necessarily limited, but it included most of those whose work was referred to in our manuscript. Among these was Dr. L. Lorand. About ten days later we received a letter from Dr. Lorand (dated April 14, 1969) pointing out that his group had previously "reported" that the factor XIII-catalyzed incorporation of dansyl cadaverine into fibrin was largely limited to the tyrosine (γ-)chain (Lorand and Tokura, unpublished observations). We immediately responded to Dr. Lorand (our letter dated May 2, 1969) assuring him that we were unaware of his findings (they had appeared only as a footnote in an article in B.B.R.C., 25, 629, 1966), and that we would certainly add a note in proof about their "unpublished data". His reply (dated May 16, 1969) was incomprehensible, and we terminated the correspondence at that point.

Our paper appeared in the June issue of PNAS and made four qualitative points:

    (a) all acceptors are on gamma-chains (we added a note about the observations of Lorand and Tokura),

    (b) there are two different kinds of crosslinked systems,

    (c) the two different systems are apparently gamma-gamma and gamma-alpha, and

    (d) beta-chains are not involved in the crosslinking process.

In addition we provided the quantitation of all these observations and suggested a detailed model of how monomeric units are arranged in fibrin polymers.

The August, 1969 issue of PNAS will evidently carry an article by Lorand and Chenoweth and communicated in May or June, 1969. In this article Lorand and Chenoweth apparently report the observations on incorporation of dansyl-cadaverine into fibrin. On August 11, 1969, a second article entitled "Chain Pairs in the Crosslinking of Fibrin" submitted under the authorship of Lorand, Chenoweth, and Domanik appeared in an October, 1969 edition of B.B.R.C. In this article the authors "discover" the following about fibrin crosslinking:

  (a) α- and γ-chains are involved in crosslinking systems.

  (b) The data are consistent with an α-γ type linkage, but the possibility of γγ and αα is noted.

  (c) Beta chains are not involved.

These conclusions are based entirely on acrylamide gel electrophoresis observations on crosslinked and non-crosslinked fibrins using a newly announced procedure (Brummal and Montgomery, in press, 1969).

In spite of the fact that these experiments were evidently conducted with full knowledge of our previous findings, there is no reference to our work nor any indication of our previous correspondence. The observations are presented in the vein of new discoveries. Not surprisingly, we didn't receive preprints of these manuscripts.

We believe very much in cooperation among groups with similar interests. Unfortunately, unilateral sharing is not a satisfactory arrangement. We trust that in the future Dr. Lorand's "oversights" will be acknowledged.

Renné Chen

R. F. Doolittle
Department of Chemistry
University of California, San Diego
La Jolla, California   92037

Addendum 4 (Chapter 7)

Laci's note to me about Russ Doolittle

NORTHWESTERN UNIVERSITY COLLEGE
OF ARTS AND SCIENCES

Section of Biological Sciences
Department of Biochemistry,
Molecular Biology, and Cell Biology

Evanston, Illinois 60201

March 23, 1983

Dr. Michael Mosesson
Department of Medicine
Mount Sinai Medical Center
950 N. 12th St.
Milwaukee, Wisc. 53233

Dear Mike:

    Thank you for phoning me. I am relieved to know that Doolittle's prevarications regarding the history for elucidating the mechanism of lobster clotting will not be printed in the Annals of the New York Academy of Sciences. For your own information, I enclose a few of our earlier reprints dealing with the subject.

    With kindest regards.

Sincerely,

Laci

L. Lorand

LL/nf

Enc .

Addendum 5 (Chapter 7)
John Finlayson's letter to me

From: John Finlayson <<rigafin@verizon.net>>
Sent: Wednesday, June 20, 2018 8:19 PM
To: 'Michael Mosesson' <<mmosesson@wi.rr.com>>
Subject: RE: Factor XIII and Lorand

Hi Guy!

  It's good to hear from you. It sounds as if you had a good time in Florida and that things are going well. Rasma and I dodder around, falling further behind in most endeavors (e.g., reading), and mostly just enjoying each other.

What I'm going to tell you is from my memory and what I have been able to lay my hands on in the last 60 minutes or so. At one point in mid- to late 1968, John Pisano wrote a long, detailed letter to Science describing the fiasco that followed our submission of the article in question (i.e., Pisano, Finlayson, & Peyton, Science 1968). Needless to say, Science never replied. I may have a copy of it, but it would be in a folder of "Fibrinogen Correspondence" in some box (of many) labeled simply "work." I will look for it, but with no guarantees of either success or a timetable.

  We submitted the article to Science in January 1968. It was received on January 19. In the letter of transmittal, which (to the best of my recollection) was brief and quite low-key, John P. asked that, in view of previously conflicting reports, the manuscript not be sent to Dr. Lorand, but stated that any other reviewers would be acceptable. Also needless to say, Science sent it to Lorand forthwith. He sat on it for months. It was eventually published on May 24, 1968. During the interval, Lorand published our results three times. Once was in an addendum to a paper in Biochemistry that was, at best, tangentially related to the subject. I believe that it was Biochemistry of March 1968, volume 7, number 3, pages 1214-1223, but I do not have a copy of it, and I could get only the first page of it through PubMed.

Another, apparently, was in the introduction to a paper in J Clinical Investigation, February 1968, volume 47, number 2, pages 268-273. In the introduction he stated that after the clotting enzyme does its thing, the remaining chains [i.e., in fibrin monomer] "...subsequently cross-link in a transpeptidating reaction to form gamma-glutamyl-epsilon-lysine bonds..." This statement is supported by the citation of three references to himself and coworkers, all of which references include H. H. Ong as one—or the only—coauthor, and all of which were published in 1966.

The third paper was the one that you apparently have, i.e., BBRC April19, volume 31, number 2, pages 222-230. I recall that John P. said at the time that there was no possible way that the experiment(s) Lorand described in that paper could have yielded the elution pattern that was shown as a figure. I wasn't sophisticated enough about peptide chromatography to make a judgement, and I haven't attempted to look up that paper.

Just to put one final bit of information in your hands, I want to mention the paper by Maticic and Loewy, which I believe was in BBRC 1968, volume 30, pages 356-362. It found exactly what Pisano et al. found, but it appeared in print much earlier. Ironically (again, if I remember correctly), it was received for publication on January 18, 1968—one day before ours. However, inasmuch as John Pisano taught Ariel Loewy the method of searching for and measuring epsilon-(gamma-glutamyl) lysine, that was no big deal. Their labs were in more-or-less constant communication.

This is all that I can think of at the minute. I'll do a little more searching of PubMed and (I hope) much more searching of those boxes (above), but as stated, no guarantees.

Addendum 6 (Chapter 7)

Letter from Laci to me, November 21, 1981

Nov. 21st, 1981

Dear Mike,

It is difficult to put in words how grateful we all are for the tremendous favour and kindness you showed, and I know I am also speaking for Michele. She is still out East; she told me on the phone that she met you in New York. All these improbable realities !!!

We are now in the process of picking up the pieces on Joyce's father. Thus far, I learnt that she served in both world wars, was 80%

disabled and wrote poetry. He was also an expert on American history. -- I came up to Milwaukee twice since I saw you, even went to the Veterans Hospital, but beside being told that there was a file on him, I could not get any details. Did you ever receive the V.A. files?

In his apartment, I found an early picture of Joyce, identical to the one we had; also some bank deposit books were handed over to me by a friend of his (the bar owner whose address he used; however, he lived elsewhere.). We would like to donate whatever money he has to honor Brian, and we are ever so grateful for the care he had there. Please convey my special thanks to

380 Hazard Street
Glencoe, Illinois 60022

the doctors and nurses in the
interview can wait. What a pity
that Joyce and Michele did not
have a chance to talk with him.

Michele and Joyce went to
see him two days after my visit.
Joyce felt he knew that she came.
We are terribly grateful for your
finding him.

Among his belongings, he
had the divorce papers from Joyce's
mother and we also found out that
he had never remarried.

What a story!

With thanks for
all you have done, Sincerely, Life

Addendum 7 (Chapter 7)

Letter from Joyce Bruner-Lorand

Dear Mike,

This brief note is just to let you know how much I appreciated all of your efforts and your kind attention afforded to my *[illegible]* during his final illness. I am most grateful to you for all these *[illegible]*, and offer my profound thanks.

Most Sincerely,

[signature]

Addendum 8 (Chapter 7)

Letter to Laci on November 4, 2009

To: Laszlo Lorand

Dear Laci:

It's good to hear from you, especially to learn that you are still actively pursuing factor XIII. I hope you and Joyce are well. I too, am still working away-lately on the a2-antiplasmin compartment that is covalently bound to circulating fibrinogen. I believe that it becomes ligated to fibrinogen while in the circulation, most likely by the action of FXIII. You may be interested in my recent article on this subject JTH 6:1565, 2008.

If by pfXIII you mean platelet derived FXIII, my understanding is that pfXIII (A2) does not bind to fibrinogen. But I guess by pfXIII you mean non-thrombin cleaved plasma factor XIII (A2B2), what I am calling FXIII. As you know, our prior observations on the binding of FXIII (A2B2) to fibrinogen showed that B subunits are required for binding to occur, and the binding is exclusively in the gamma prime chains. However, A subunits may contribute to that binding, but alone they do not bind to fibrinogen-or at least too weakly for me to demonstrate binding.

In that regard, I want to caution you about the seriously flawed experiments reported by Moaddel, Farrell, et al. a few years ago on binding of FXIII to fibrinogen (Biochemistry 39:6698, 2000), but you probably already know this. They did not realize that FXIII is an active enzyme when calcium ions are included in an incubation mixture with fibrinogen, and they concluded incorrectly that FXIII binds non-covalently to both gA and g' fibrinogen. In fact, FXIII-mediated ligation was occurring under their experimental conditions. I can discuss this further with you if you wish, but I think I have said enough on this subject. [*italics* mine]

We tried to purify B subunits at the time of our binding experiments, and it was very difficult for us to obtain solutions of B subunits that behave the way we wanted them to, so we were not able to follow up in studying B subunit binding to fibrinogen. In the presence of purified B subunits, fibrinogen kept precipitating. Kevin Siebenlist and I finally gave up. Good luck if you wish to try that.

As far as stoichiometry is concerned, what we do know is that virtually all the factor XIII activity in human plasma is bound to fibrinogen, and that to purify FXIII from plasma, one must first heat denature the fibrinogen to release the FXIII that is bound. You yourself adequately demonstrated that in your published method for purifying FXIII from plasma, which we still use. We have taken it a bit further and shown that FXIII from our murine human g'-fibrinogen mouse, or for that matter wild-type mice, is bound to the murine fibrinogen. Moreover, purification of murine FXIII follows the same purification pathway as human.

I hope this information is useful to you. We really should get together soon for lunch or dinner. We are not far from one another. Best wishes, Michael

Addendum 9 (Chapter 7)

Letters from Laci to me and my response

November 10, 2009 (Email)

Dear Mike: I could not thank you earlier, because Joyce was hospitalized with--from the cytology of ascites--seems to be ovarian ca. CAT scans show no abnormality. This is as bad as it gets. The info you gave me is exactly what I needed; since this is for a chapter I am writing, I would be grateful if you could give me the best relevant 2-3 refs. In regard of nomenclature, I try to follow the Ariens et al study group guidelines which are pretty much what I was using anyway.----May I ask a few more clarifications. 1) Is there evidence that B stays with the polymerizing fibrin after A is dissociated from it. In other words, plasma B vs serum B concentration? I suggested somewhere that B was modified to B' by A*, but did not follow up on that. 2) I long entertained the notion that dimeric fibrinogen (we always see some in plasma) might represent the small fraction of the clotting protein that carries AB; perhaps these are gamma' dimers???? 3) Is there good evidence that the actual act of crosslinking of a2PI --as compared to its very tight non-covalent association with fibrin-- was essential for endowing the clot to resist fibrinolysis?--Would you be good enough to help me whatever ref I should quote.----Would be a pleasure to see you. Let's hope we can get together. Laci

November 13, 2009 (Email)

To: Mosesson, Michael Subject: Re: fXIII, FXIII, pfXIII, etc.

I sent this off without finishing my questions, Mike. The TH article with Pat McKee would seem to imply that thrombin was activated in blood all the time and that the activation of fXIII took precedence over the reaction of thrombin with fibrinogen, i.e., production of fibrin (is there continuous clot formation; does fibrinogen turn over as fibrin; is there a steady state for FPA release?). Furthermore, it implies that there should be significant fXIIIa transamidating activity in plasma. Am I correct in these assumptions??-Can one exclude that the incorporation of a2PI is not catalyzed by whatever TG2 activity may be discharged into plasma (by hemolysis)?

Dear Laci:

I'm saddened to hear about Joyce's cytology report. I hope there is some treatment that can be used to cure her or to mitigate her ascites. And yes, we should all get together soon. You name the time and the place.

As far as the second part of your message, re: the TH article with Pat McKee, that article did not imply or infer that thrombin is activated in blood all the time or even at all. What was shown in that work is that FXIII is active in the presence of calcium ions with respect to substrates like fibrinogen and a2AP. In fact, it would not be correct to infer that thrombin plays any role in the incorporation of a2AP into fibrinogen in the circulation. Where would it come from? How could thrombin exist in any appreciable amounts without leading at the same time to fibrin formation? As previously shown by Kevin and me (TH 86:1221, 2001), FXIII (without activation by thrombin) is inactive when it comes to DNScad incorporation into casein, but under the same solvent conditions it can by itself ligate fibrinogen or fibrin, just as thrombin activated FXIIIa does, and almost as rapidly. It seems possible that incorporation of a2AP into fibrinogen in blood might be catalyzed by TG2, as you state, but there is by now definitive proof that FXIII can itself catalyze such incorporation. I know about RBC TG2 and the possibility of hemolysis, but why conjure up an alternative explanation for an activity that is already there?

As for your other questions, 1) I'm not sure whether B subunits stay with polymerizing fibrin after A dissociates. 2) I don't have any information on the composition of fibrinogen dimers, nor whether they carry AB as a feature. A few years ago, with the help of *Jim Hainfeld* and *Joe Wall* at the Brookhaven STEM facility, we showed that non-covalently linked fibrinogen dimers existed, apparently owing to a moderate tendency for self-association of the fibrinogen D domains (Mosesson et al. J Struct Biol 115:88, 1995). 3) The question about whether a2AP bound to fibrinogen confers resistance against fibrinolysis is a good one. I believe that it does. Believe it or not, I found evidence for that effect as a neophyte at the very beginning of my research career (J Clin Invest 42:747, 1963). The reason I am still doing research these days is to address that very question. 4) The association between a2AP and fibrinogen is covalent for several reasons, the most important one being that it is not dissociable from the fibrinogen Aa chains under reducing conditions.

I'm not sure which specific references to send you because I do not know the complete context of your request. If you want references relating to the binding of FXIII to fibrinogen g' chains, you already know them all. *And I caution you again about citing the data and conclusions provided by Moaddel et al. in 2000 (Biochemistry 39:6698, 2000). [italics mine]* I also can refer you to a very recent review by Shirley Uitte de Willige in Blood (114:3994, 2009). Shirley is a highly competent investigator as far as haplotypes and clinical thrombosis are concerned, but she is out of her element when it comes to understanding FXIII and fibrinogen. Note that she has uncritically cited the Moadell article in her discussion of FXIII binding to fibrinogen. Other authors have repeatedly cited this work, including Dave Farrell himself, but consensus does not represent evidence, as you well know.

So there we are my old friend. You have stimulated quite a detailed response from me, and I restate that am willing to help you in any way that I can. Remember the episode at Sinai Samaritan Hospital in 1983 that involved Joyce's father, your daughter, Michele, and you yourself? I bring this up now only to convey my recollections and fondness for Joyce, and for you. I sincerely hope we continue this dialogue and that we can get together sometime soon. Michael

Scanning Transmission Electron Microscopy (STEM)

Many experiments related to the fibrin cross-linking issue were carried out at the Brookhaven National Laboratory (BNL) Scanning Transmission Electron Microscope (STEM) Facility headed by *Joseph Wall* who had advanced this powerful imaging technology for the study of biological specimens. Following my introduction to this subject in 1979, I spent more than twenty years as a frequent BNL visitor to study a multitude of issues mainly concerned with fibrinogen and fibrin structure, a profitable collaboration that lasted beyond 2002. My work at BNL began with a study of fibrinogen structure and the location of the domains comprising each molecule, using STEM imaging coupled with mass analyses of objects in the fields of view. I reviewed that experience in Chapter V of *Fibrinogen Memoirs* [1]. The report that emerged was the first of many to follow that utilized STEM to obtain high resolution images of proteins and carry out mass analyses of objects that had been imaged. In addition to studies of Fibrinogen and Fibrin using STEM, I also successfully investigated several blood proteins including Blood Clotting Factor V (with *Mike Nesheim*), Factor VIII (with *Pete Lollar*), and Factor XIII, von Willebrand Factor, Fibronectin, and α2-Antiplasmin.

STEM has important qualitative and quantitative advantages over Transmission Electron Microscopy (TEM). STEM specimens do not require the addition of electron dense contrasting agents or metal shadowing procedures to define their shapes and interactions, and they are processed in volatile solvents resulting in specimens that are salt-free after freeze-drying under high vacuum for subsequent imaging. Images are obtained on the basis of a specimen's capacity to scatter an incident 40 kV electron beam of sufficiently low intensity to assure minimal radiation damage. Scattered electrons are processed to produce a digitized image of the 'native' protein. Since the electron beam is focused at 0.25 nm, the obtainable resolution is much higher than is possible with TEM, which requires the addition of electron dense contrasting solutions or metal shadowing for visualizing specimens. For one example, we used the high resolution obtainable with STEM to image gold-tagged (3 nm particle) carboxy-terminal regions of γ chains in fibrinogen molecules and in assembled fibrin fibrils [19].

STEM Mass Analysis–A Powerful Tool

The *mass* of an object imaged by STEM is proportional to the number of scattered electrons. Processing of these scattered electrons yields high resolution digitized STEM images. These images can be further processed offline by a *mass analysis* program. We used a 'fiber program' to compute mass per unit length of fibrin fibrils, as illustrated below. Since the molecular weight of fibrin is known (340 kD), the value for mass per unit length can unambiguously indicate the number of strands in a fibril or in each arm of a branch junction (**Figure**).

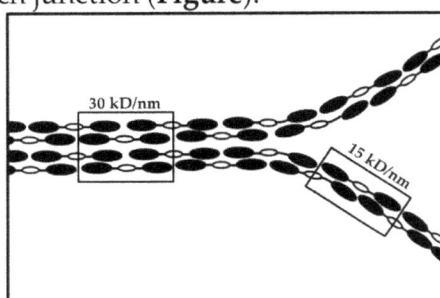

Figure. *A drawing of two double-stranded fibrils, each fibril composed of a half staggered linear array of fibrin molecules, each one 45 nm in length* ●━○━● *with a mass of 340 kD. The rectangular field enclosing a two-stranded fibril would yield a mass per unit length of 15 kD/nm, whereas a four-stranded fibril would yield twice that value, 30 kD/nm. Reproduced from Reference [1].*

Mass analysis of objects from a STEM image is a versatile and powerful tool that has been used as described above and in other ways. For example, we used mass analyses to identify cross-linked D-fibrin-D ●●●● complexes based upon its predicted mass [12] (Chapter 8).

In our investigation of cross-linked fibrinogen fibrils [13] (Chapter 10) we obtained high resolution STEM images of the fibrils and other related structures that enabled us to identify the filaments representing cross-linked γ chains that extended *transversely* from one fibril strand to the other. These determinations were supplemented by mass analyses of substructures whenever appropriate. We also used STEM mass analysis for the same purposes in investigating fibrils that formed on a Fragment E template [18] (Chapter 12). STEM analyses described in this document offered unassailable evidence for a *transverse* cross-linking arrangement and added more heft to other already published evidence pointing in that same direction.

Acknowledgements

My sincerest gratitude to *Leonid Medved* for his constructive suggestions and wise counsel during manuscript preparation. I also wish to acknowledge the seminal reports from *Eberhard Selmayr*. These contributions aroused my long-term interest in verifying his exposition of the location of cross-linked γ chains in fibrin fibrils. I again acknowledge the contributions of *John Ferry*. His prior investigations, coupled with his insightful correspondence, revealed to me the ineluctable relationship between *fibrin elasticity* and *transverse* positioning of γ chain cross-links. I thank *Roger Chen* for his artful caricatures of the participants in the controversy. These drawings add spice and insight into each person's character and disposition. I also thank *Libby Temkin* for her insightful suggestions on phraseology and content; and *Lisa Roma* for her artful and precise editing and layout design of this second volume of Fibrinogen Memoirs.

Names Cited

Ariens, Robert

Belitser, Vladimir

Bishop, Paul

Blombäck, Birger

Bruner, Robert

Bruner-Lorand, Joyce

Budzynski, Andrei

Chenoweth, D

Cohen, Carolyn

Cohn, EJ

DiOrio, Jim

Domanik, RA

Doolittle, Russell

Duval, Cedric

Ferry, John

Finlayson, John

Fowler, Walter

Guthold, Martin

Hainfeld, James

Henschen, Agnes

Ingham, Ken

Koenderink, GH

Kumiawan, NA

Laki, Koloman

Landel, Robert

Litvinov, Rustem

Loewy, Ariel

Lollar, Pete

Lorand, Lazlo

Lorand, Michele

Lord, Susan

Lottspeich, F.

Maeterlinck, Maurice

Marder, Victor

Matiçic, S.

McKee, Patrick

Medved, Leonid

Morrison, Peter

Mosesson, Michael

Müller-Berghaus, Gert

Nesheim, Mike

Oncley, J. Laurence

Peyton, Marjorie

Pierchocka, IK

Pisano, John

Privalov, Peter

Rocco, Mattia

Schrag, John

Selmayr, Eberhard

Siebenlist, Kevin

Szent-Györgyi, Albert

Veklich, Yuri

Vos, BA

Wall, Joseph

Weisel, John

Yakovlev, Sergei

Zhmurov, Artemis

www.ingramcontent.com/pod-product-compliance
Lightning Source LLC
Chambersburg PA
CBHW052338210326
41597CB00031B/5295